A BLIND HOG'S ACORNS

A Blind Hog's Acorns

Vignettes of the Maladies of Workers

by

CARRY P. McCORD, M.D.

With Illustrations by Strobel

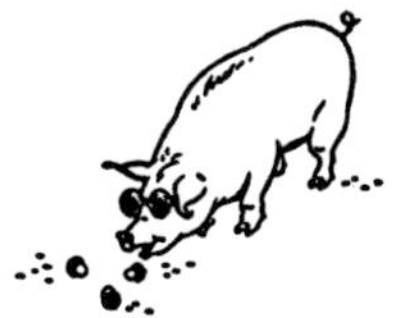

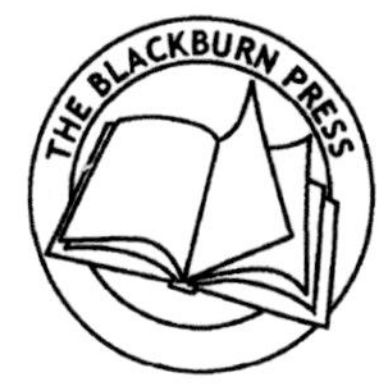

Reprint of First Edition 1945, Cloud, Inc.

A Blind Hog's Acorns

ISBN-10: 1-930665-20-2
ISBN-13: 978-1-930665-20-0

Library of Congress Control Number: 00-2001088257

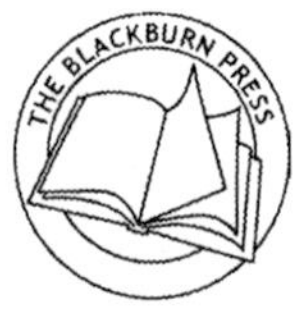

THE BLACKBURN PRESS
P. O. Box 287
Caldwell, New Jersey 07006 U.S.A.
973-228-7077
www.BlackburnPress.com

To

The Scores of Associates

Who Have Come, Gone and Stayed

During the Past Twenty-Five Years,

and in Particular

To

The Then

D.K.M.

Foreword to 2001 Reprinting

Cary Pratt McCord was a simple Alabama country boy who early in life had the misfortune of being diagnosed by an itinerant phrenologist as having the intellect of a blind hog. His worried parents, however, were consoled by being told that "even a blind hog gets an acorn once in a while;" This mis-labeling had a profound impact upon his relationship with people and, subsequently, with the world. During his formative years, he shunned the company of people and displayed a consuming interest in things: rocks, plants, trees, chemicals and, above all, books. Accompanying his father, a crusading Baptist minister who could find sin to fight in the neighboring mining camps, sawmills and cotton mill towns, he was exposed to a variety of new work-related problems (e.g., brushes with mine disasters such as fire, black, or stink damp, cotton mill workers and their "asthma", the crude distillation of tars and pitch in lumber camps)--all of these stoked his abiding curiosity in the ills of the workplace.

Despite the phrenologic misdiagnosis, he managed to graduate from primary and high schools and from college. While working in a coal mine, he was accepted by the medical school in Ann Arbor Michigan, where, given his proclivity for "things," he gravitated toward laboratory medicine. After graduation in 1912, he spent several years in endocrine research, taking his first postgraduate job as research physiologist at Parke-Davis, the pharmaceutical manufacturer. This was followed by a stint as a Colonel in the Army Medical Corps during World War I. There, he met Christian R. Holmes, Dean of the Medical College of the University of Cincinnati, who nourished his growing interest in health problems related to environmental exposures and, in 1918, invited him to come to Cincinnati to help start a School of Public Health. Unfortunately, Dr. Holmes disappeared in the Arctic while on a post-war expedition and the school never materialized. Left at a loose end, Dr. McCord continued to expand his knowledge of the workplace and the world of work, and to hone his skills in the use of such simple industrial hygiene environmental measurement tools as were then available.

In 1920, he created the Industrial Health Conservancy Laboratories to serve as a home for his independent animal research as well as a base for his burgeoning activity as a consultant. He was called on by industries, labor unions, local, state and federal governmental agencies and served frequently as an expert witness in cases of litigation over injuries and illnesses attributed to workplace hazards. The laboratory was moved from Cincinnati to Detroit where he first served as Professor of Occupational Diseases at Wayne State University and then joined the faculty of the University of Michigan School of Public Health in Ann Arbor. He not only organized and directed the industrial hygiene program of the local health department but also organized and directed the Industrial Hygiene Department of the State of Michigan.

In 1935, while continuing to respond to the increasing demand for his services as a consultant and as an expert witness in medico-legal cases, he became *de facto* Medical Director of the Chrysler Corporation and led the effort to control the lead poisoning that was then highly prevalent in the automotive industry. His experiences were promptly shared with colleagues through lectures and journal articles; during his professional life, he was credited with thousands of published articles and more than a dozen books.

He became widely known for the excellence and clarity of his lectures and presentations and for his skill as a moderator. At the same time, however, he was disliked by many for his intensity, his seeming aloofness and, above all, the acerbic wit with which he attacked what he saw as laziness, stupidity and lack of integrity. He was a superb teacher and mentor, devoting much time and energy to pushing his younger associates ahead as long as they had ability and were willing to work hard.

The publication of *A Blind Hog's Acorns* in 1945--and the acclaim with which it was received (it rapidly went through several printings)--represented something of an epiphany in Dr. McCord's persona. It was not so much that he had changed, as those who worked closely with him and knew him well could testify. Rather, it was the change from the perception of him by many as an intense, hard-driving, ambitious, demanding, self-centered "genius" to the recognition of the humane, caring, perceptive and really friendly individual he always had been.

Perhaps it was the mellowing of aging--he was 60 when this appeared (he lived to the ripe old age of 93)--and the realization of the magnitude of his accomplishments over the years. In addition to his scientific and scholarly contributions, he played leading roles in the Industrial Medical Association, the Industrial Hygiene Association, the American Academy of Occupational Medicine and other professional organizations. He served as editor of *Industrial Medicine and Surgery* and later of the *Journal of Occupational Medicine* and, in 1947, he received the coveted Knudsen Award, bestowed by the American Occupational Medical Association (now the American College of Occupational and Environmental Medicine) in recognition of a lifetime of accomplishment in the field. In any case, he seemed to relax and, reversing the focus of his youth, began to display more interest in people than in things.

He became something of a "character." When attending national medical meetings, for example, he would settle in a chair near the elevators in the lobby of the headquarters hotel. There, he would hold court chatting with contemporaries and younger colleagues who recognized him while making their way to the sessions.

He organized, and largely directed, the annual invitational Selby Conferences at the University of Michigan. These were attended by some 40 or 50 leaders in the field of occupational medicine who came from around the country to spend several days in an informal exchange of ideas and experiences and getting previews of the latest in research. The highlight of these meetings was the annual session chaired by Dr. McCord in which he good-naturedly alternately wheedled and needled attendees into expressing their thoughts on current issues of controversy. The luckiest were those who arrived in Ann Arbor early enough to be invited to the "open house" in Dr. McCord's home or had a seat at his table for the annual dinner session.

A Blind Hog's Acorns is a delightful compendium of anecdotes. Written in an unassuming style reminiscent of the "oral histories" being collected by the Library of Congress, they offer charming vignettes of interesting people, places and events. Who can forget the startling and starkly limned images of the "big city" consultant, accompanied by two frostbitten secretaries, pumping a railroad handcar through a snowstorm to reach an assignment? Of Jake Fulsome, the night pottery kiln fireman who, while "under the influence," discovered a new and marvelous way of manufacturing a unique vase while almost burning down the kiln? And of Junius, the brilliant but alcoholic doctor whose ministrations brought comfort to the rural poor and the forgotten in the hill country?

But the book is more than that. In the aggregate, the anecdotes present an engaging history of the beginnings of the disciplines of occupational medicine and industrial hygiene in the United States. The reader is left with a rich comprehension of the harsh realities of the period of American industrial development between 1920 and 1935 and the pain experienced by the workers on the lowest rungs of society's ladder, especially those who were left behind as a legacy of racism and the provincialism of rural backwaters. It is indeed a classic!

Bertram D. Dinman, MD, ScD*

August 8, 2000

*Dr. Dinman is Clinical Professor of Occupational Medicine at the University of Pittsburgh School of Public Health. He had been successively Corporate Medical Director and Vice President-Health and Safety of the Aluminum Corporation of America. Earlier, he spent a decade with Dr. McCord on the faculty of the University of Michigan School of Public Health. Like Dr. McCord, he is a recipient of the Knudsen Award from the American College of Occupational and Environmental Medicine.

Contents

Chapter

1. The Coming of the Phrenologist 1
2. What Are the Hazardous Trades? 8
3. Getting Ready for the Hazardous Trades 17
4. The First Job 30
5. Hannah's Hand 36
6. Dust is a Friend and a Foe 44
7. Trial by Dust 50
8. Two Ghosts of a City 59
9. Amateur Versus Expert Pottery Making 70
10. Jungle Ulcer 77
11. A Little Piece of Man 96
12. Coroner for a Day 99
13. Panic 105
14. My Boss 111
15. The Offensive Trades 119
16. Chlorine and Chicanery 127
17. The Four O'Clock Mystery 135
18. Women at Work 141
19. The Man Who Refused to be Poisoned 150
20. Medical Sideshow 156

21. The Tale of Two Coats 162
22. Saving the Surface 171
23. Threats from the Refrigerator 178
24. Dancing Eyes 185
25. Journey to Junius 191
26. The Doctor and the Rabbi 199
27. Hammer Head 203
28. A Minor Medical Miracle 208
29. The Birth of the B. A. 213
30. A Reversal in Diagnosis 220
31. Little Giants 226
32. Black Turns White 231
33. La Maladie de Skevos Zervos 237
34. Arsenicism 241
35. Blindness from Benzol 247
36. Metal Fever 250
37. The Country Doctor Shows Up the Expert 257
38. Fits from the Furnace 264
39. The Workers' Crotchets and Incubuses 272
40. Uncle Jeff's Big Catch 282
41. "Tet" and "Tri" 289
42. The Preferred Professions 295
43. Chrysanthemums' Fingerprints 301
44. This Amazing Present 307

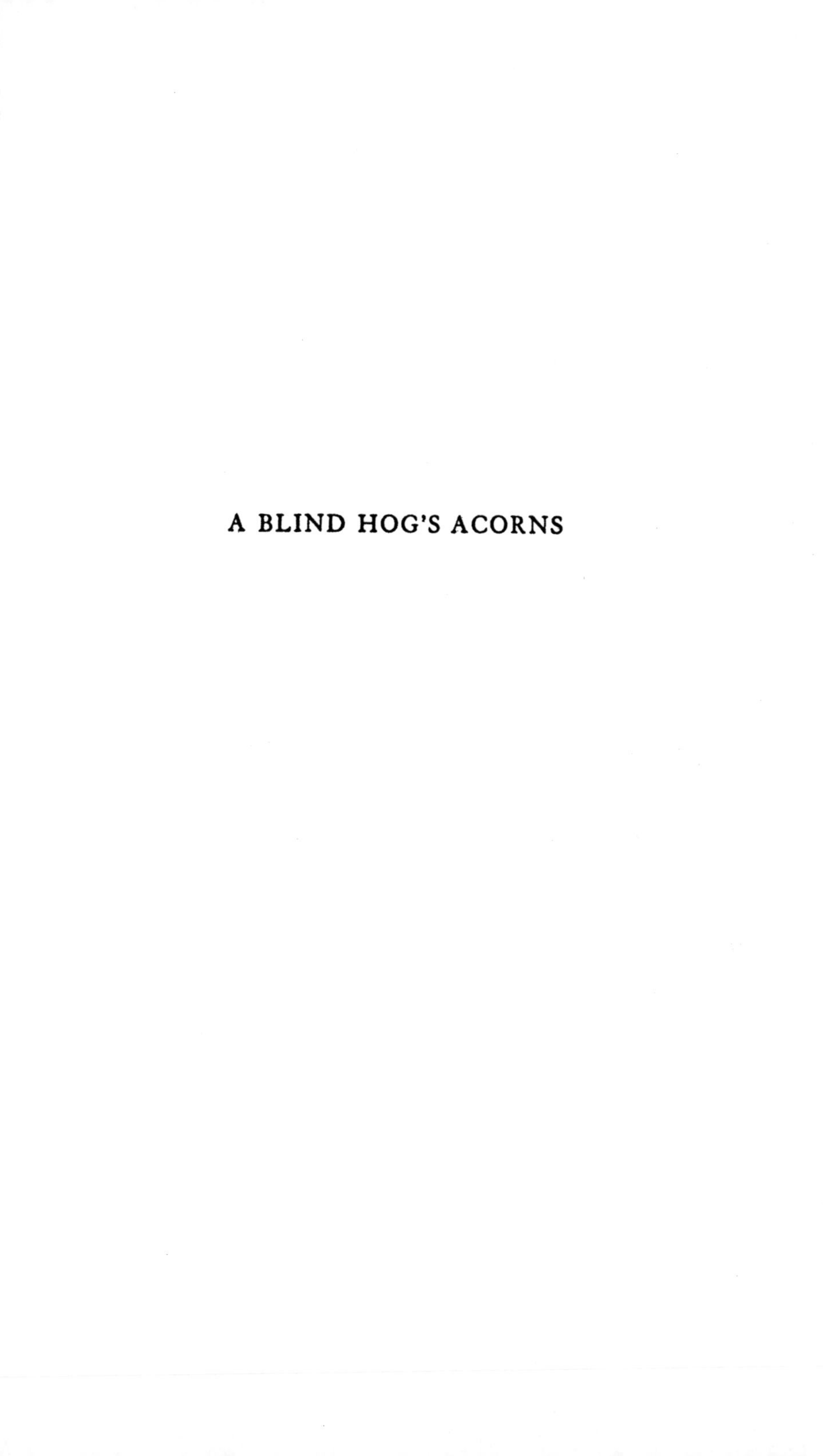

A BLIND HOG'S ACORNS

Chapter I

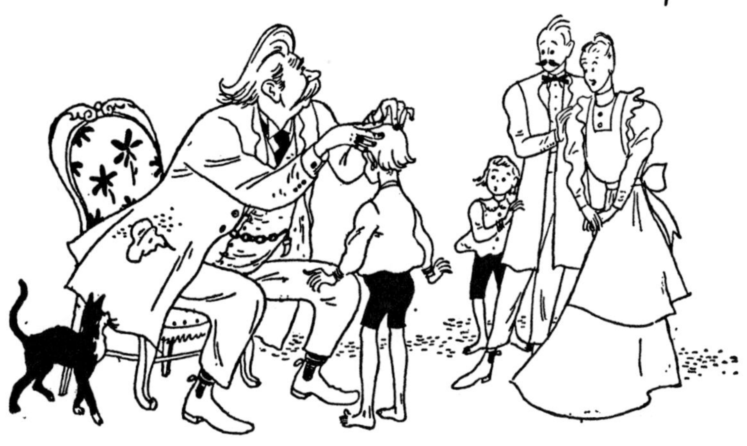

The Coming of the Phrenologist

FIFTY years ago and more in the towns of Alabama, the homes of preachers served as substitutes for hotels. "Drummers," peddlers, horse traders, farmers, missionaries, caught in the town at night regularly expected the preacher to live up to Biblical injunctions, and he did.

Our house at least weekly sheltered a transient. His horse got the stall while ours was left out on the "patch." He got the best bed, and some of the family slept on pallets.

In the house of the preacher every traveller-sinner became a saint. "Brother" and "Sister" embellished his conversation as obvious, if temporary, evidence of his devoutness. Sometimes, however, he tendered his wares in honest payment — the shoe salesman, a pair of cheap shoes; the peddler, a few yards of lace; occasionally a farmer brought a real prize, a shoat, most often the runt; the bookseller always left a Bible — but we had so many Bibles. We wanted other books but seldom got them. The itinerant dentists were the worst.

They insisted on doing a little work, even when it was not needed. To this day I bear the evidence of half-quack dental lodging payments.

One night the phrenologist came — with pudginess, a walrus mustache and pomposity. My father fully accepted the great man of science and his jargon. In those days when a fat man had a little buggy which he nearly overfilled, and a little horse to go with it, it was a bad sign. In the case of the phrenologist, my father was so pleased to have such a distinguished guest that he overlooked the warning.

Next morning the great man offered to read the heads of the preacher's two boys. This would pay for everything; moreover, it would establish the phrenologist in the community. I, being five at the time, was the elder; my brother was four. Later there were other children, but they escaped the head reading business. My head was pushed, squeezed and measured. Soon the phrenologist muttered to himself, sighed, gasped. He was exasperated. This wasn't going to make for good business in our town.

At the end he spoke in pain, still pontifically, but without the language of the pontiff, "Brother and Sister, I can't understand how a boy with a head like this got in your family. His bumps are all wrong." Mother looked startled. "He won't be able to take much schoolin', and it might kill him if you pushed him." I was being regarded in mute horror. "His intellect," the wise man elaborated, "is about like one of these Alabama blind hogs. His head proves he just ain't fittin'." Looking up to the faces of my stricken parents, he was apparently moved to soften the blow. "Of course," he consoled, "even a blind hog gets an acorn once in a while."

My brother fared better. He was held out as the hope of the family. It seemed that wherever my head was in intaglio, his was in rilievo, and vice versa. At four, he accepted his triumph with all the concern of a winner of a turtle derby. Not so my parents. My father, in deep religious conviction, took the stand.

"Even if he hasn't much sense, he has a soul that might be lost to Hell. I, as his father, will make every effort to assure that his soul is saved. Maybe he will fare better in Heaven." My mother, no less affected, accepted the monster as her own.

Thereafter for many months, the chief topic of conversation among kith, kin, neighbors, visitors and strangers was the baleful misfortune that had befallen our family. Several times a week demonstrations were given of the very spots where there were no brains. To any who may be seeking methods of inflicting psychic trauma, this method is highly commended.

Then began a boyhood devoted to "things," or, negatively, to the shunning of people. For one saddled with the stigma of not being "fittin'" it seemed quite necessary, lazar-like, to keep away from others who were.

A continuous household alert was established. Every gate was made to squeak loudly, announcing the approach of any outsider. There were many hideouts—chiefly the privy where one's presence might appear reasonable, at least for a time, or the flower pit if one were caught on the other side of the house. In winter it was possible to burrow into the cottonseed hulls in the cow barn. Ways were found to cover the distance from our house on the outskirts to the business district by following alleys and cutting across vacant lots. Not a person was likely to be seen until the store or post office was reached.

A few human contacts proved inescapable. These few caused horripilation (since no medical dictionary is beside you—just plain goose pimples). Once the passing of the town's nabob on a narrow path became inevitable. As I came near, he properly turned out to his right. I darted to my left,—an impasse. He then tried his left. I tried my right,—a collision. We repeated several times until in exasperation, he said, "Boy, if you will just stand still, I will go around you." I did, and he did, but my flesh still quivers at the memory of that encounter.

There were many "things" to provide interests—rocks, trees, plants, insects, animals, chemicals, books. A crusading Baptist preacher in those days never would be content to stay long in any one place. Always there was more sin in some other town — mining camps, sawmill towns, cottonmill towns. The last were the worst. In moving from one town to another in wagons, it was customary merely to tie the chickens' legs together, thus making them helpless, and toss them onto the loaded wagon. Of us it was said that our chickens were so accustomed to moving that whenever a wagon stopped before our gate, the chickens lay down and crossed their legs waiting to be tied. We moved, moved, moved.

This was fortunate, for it meant more new "things." At one time we lived immediately above the entrance to the "diggings,"— a coal mine. The continual noise must have been at about the ninety decibel level, but no one seemed to notice.

One day there was excitement. "Black damp" had gotten into the mine — men were dead. At the mine entrance, a hushed, awed, resentful crowd gathered, waiting the bringing up of the bodies to the surface. Most of all I wanted to know what "black damp" might be, but I didn't have the courage to ask. Someone else did. "It is a poisonous mine gas," a spokesman replied, and continued, "There are all sorts of damps —'white damp,' 'fire damp,' 'stink damp.' "

Not until many years later did I learn that in the vernacular of the miner, "black damp" is carbon dioxide, a simple asphyxiant; "white damp" is carbon monoxide, a treacherous poison; "stink damp" is hydrogen sulfide, a deadly intoxicant; "fire damp" is methane, a highly inflammable gas.

At other "diggings" there were "gob" piles and "gob" fires. At most coal mines there is much slate and other rock representing the "over" and "under" burden of the coal seam. Hauled out, it becomes miniature man-made mountains in the vicinity. There is always some coal mixed with the slate, and, in time, spontaneous combustion leads to slow-burning fires that may last for years. I saw that downwind from these fires, gases killed all vegetation. There was little white paint on any residences, but that little soon turned slaty black. The miners' families complained that their few pieces of silver were tarnished, that clocks wouldn't run, that chickens wouldn't lay, that everyone had "asthma," that washed clothes rotted on the line. The miners found solace in "mule kick" whiskey. The women lay siege to my father, the community voice of protest. All this I recorded in a near-subconscious log of things that seemed to be wrong.

As one part of my father's pastoral wanderings we found ourselves in the area of "wood coalings"—the making of charcoal. Vast amounts of small pine timbers were heaped into sizable earth-covered pyramids and fired. Slow burning produced charcoal. Now and again, some workman in recovering the charcoal would drop in his tracks wholly unconscious. Occasionally one died. All manner of explanations were offered and fantastic preventive measures introduced. Today any eighth grade pupil might point out that incomplete combustion provided carbon monoxide. The world of that far gone day was not one of chemistry but of the supernatural.

At one of the numerous schools—at times a different school for every grade—the liquor-thirsty negro janitor with a little learning, painfully spelled out "alcohol" on one of the makeshift laboratory bottles. He drank anything. This was "methyl alcohol"—wood alcohol, and soon his horrible screams upset the school and the community. The town's doctor did futile things. The janitor died. A new item was added to the log.

By this time it had become apparent that where there were interesting "things" there were apt to be people. Slowly it became a little easier to accept people.

On the outside of a woodworking mill where axe handles were shaped, a small crowd gathered. I braved the crowd and learned that the local doctor was ministering to a workman who had caught the ends of his fingers under a "sander." Some flesh had been ground off but the nails were intact. The well-meaning doctor, perhaps blessed only with the lowest of surgical judgment, announced with finality, "You won't ever heal up so long as you have your nails. They are poison. I am going to pull them out." This he proceeded to do without antisepsis, without anesthesia, without allowing the patient even to sit. His instrument was a pair of unsterile factory pliers. Rarely have I ever seen greater human suffering.

In the mind of a shambling boy, all these things, and more like them, created the deep conviction that "Work is dangerous, and doctors don't know enough about workers and work dangers."

It may not be said that I then and there determined to do something about these wrongs; but some seeds were being sown, and those seeds were unrecognized acorns.

Tangible acorns were rare. When I was about twelve, a wonderful thing happened. An agent for a traveling library endeavoring to establish a paying branch in our town of that year, with ostentation and loudness so that all might know, presented me with the first membership. Mine was free, free, free. This was an honor. No other person had one. This was recognition. Of course, I did not analyze to the point of knowing that the agent quite openly was attempting to gain my father's abetment. I am glad I had no such awareness. Without any blasphemous implications, I know that this not wholly guileless stranger came nearer saving my soul than some others seeking to apply more direct and more churchlike methods.

Following the commands of the phrenologist, the blind hog was given such schooling as he could take. Through some miracle the grades were passed, the equivalent of high school, then college, university. One day I found myself a physician, graduated, licensed. Of course, the yokedom of "things" determined that at first as a physician I belonged to the laboratory. Laboratory medicine, unfortunately, all too frequently embraces services apart from the patient.

Many years later, at a time when a college graciously gave me an honorary degree of "Doctor of Laws," conferred, I hope, solely because of services to industry with its workers in the fields of occupational diseases and industrial hygiene — the hazardous trades —

my charming and beaming mother was near me. There were the usual pageantry, color, ceremonies, laudations. After a while the crowds went away and the two of us were alone. Without any real uncertainty, but with a little playfully assumed confusion, she said, "Maybe the phrenologist was wrong after all."

"No, not all," I said. "I think he has proved his point. You remember, he did concede the possibility of a few acorns."

"But," she continued, and with parental bias, "there have been so many acorns. Acres of acorns."

This, then, becomes a record of some professional acorns. Not all are from the same tree or of the same size. Possibly, too, not all are in the same state of preservation.

Chapter 2

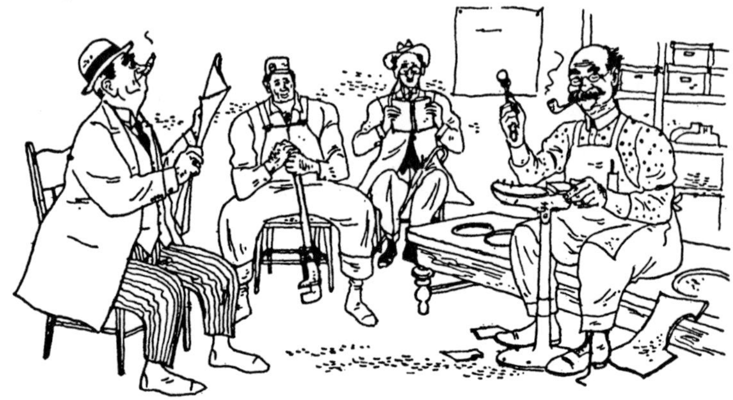

What Are the Hazardous Trades?

"THE eagle soars before she shrieks." With such a precedent, before any outpouring of one physician's adventures with the strange diseases of the workaday world, it may be advantageous to delay the recounting of happenings long enough to soar over the world of work in its entirety, and to survey the background from which derive a lot of wholly unwanted industrial by-products— trade diseases, industrial diseases, occupational diseases. These sometimes are called the "echeoses"— diseases from work.

At once there must be shared the fact that work is saddled with a lot of meaningless terms which thoroughly promote confusion.

Just what constitutes a trade, a craft, personal service, a job, a profession?

What is meant by industry, trade, manufacturing, commerce, merchandising?

There was a time when it was conceived that if a person worked with his hands and apparently without the necessity of thinking, he was a tradesman, or craftsman, or artisan. Far down the scale, he might have been termed a laborer. At the upper-crust of work, some favored persons were deemed to function in occupations characterized chiefly by thinking and not by manual toil. Such occupations were put into the category of professions. A few professions were given still higher status by the designation "learned"—law, theology, and medicine.

Any attempt now to apply this line of demarcation is doomed to defeat.

Much of modern industry so uses automatic machinery that the former tradesmen, craftsmen, or artisans have been transformed into machine tenders. By this process they are not necessarily moved upward into the professions with the disappearance of the need for work by hand, but it is granted that some degree of thinking is requisite to the tending of machines. Professional men would resent any implication that they merely sit and think. While every movement of the surgeon's hands must be governed by thought, foremostly he is a manual worker. More so is the dentist, the artist, and possibly the architect. Conceding, as will all, that there are obvious differences in the level of work of the sewer cleaner and the university president, it may be recognized that midway between is a stratum of work defying classification. The chiropodist stoutly may assert his participation in a highly skilled profession. Many feet, if articulate, would agree, but the banker might not be willing to move over and make room for the chiropodist in any assemblage of his peers.

My good shoemaker hung out the sign in front of his place of business, "Dr. C. F. Jones." When asked of what he was a doctor and where he acquired his degree, he announced, "I am the best shoemaker in this city. I am the head of my profession of shoe repairing, and I gave myself the degree." His position is here unassailed. Perhaps the best shoemaker possesses more professional attributes than the lowermost lawyer — if lawyers are here offended, substitute "physician."

Since this is a pleasant book, ungiven to controversy, no effort will be made to construct a cabinet with a top drawer assigned to preferred professions, a bottom drawer for the crafts and trades, and a middle drawer for all other forms of work. Instead, one large drawer is here created for all workers. This drawer is labeled "Occupations."

The same sort of analysis applied to such terms as "industry," "business," "commerce," "manufacturing" will lead to an equal realization of the lack of well-defined boundaries. The telephone operator would resent any classification that marks her as an industrial worker. But, is it not true that she renders helpful services in the communications industry? It seldom occurs to the salesman in a department store that he is part of the merchandising industry. The purser on a Great Lakes passenger steamer wears a uniform and thinks of himself as a sailor, but is he not in fact an indispensable unit in the transportation industry? A highly skilled attorney may align himself with an industrial corporation and render services on the plant premises, but thereby he does not lose his status as a lawyer.

Deep-rooted custom limits the term "industry" to manufacturing, mining, and transportation. Without obvious reason, this triad is set apart from scores of others such as the agricultural industry, the construction industry, the communications industry. Recourse to dictionaries and encyclopedias affords no splints for muddled minds. These books are likewise muddled. Someone must rewrite them. But it is not the function of this book to essay any confusion-dispelling terminology. Instead, the confusion merely is recognized, and an attempt will be made to live with it. In order that there may be some low common denominator, all employments are simply designated as "work," all persons involved therein as "workers," and their different forms of work as "occupations."

Under any name, toil with its endless variety of machines, materials, and methods may lead to a profusion of strange diseases among workers. Manifestly, some trades are more dangerous than others. Some introduce hazards for all persons plying them. With few exceptions, all may be carried out in such fashion as to be dangerous to some workers.

Across my desk sat a pessimistic chemist who stated, "Everything used in industry with the exception of rain water may be harmful." I dissent from both of the major portions of his statement. There are indeed many substances manipulated in the world of work that do not cause injury, and, conversely, even water long in contact with the human body may lead to damage.

Long ago, Ramazzini, the patron saint of industrial hygiene, observed that in attempting to diagnose a condition in any ailing workman, the most significant question to be asked was, "Of what trade is he?" A sort of millennium for the industrial hygienist will have evolved when applicants for jobs in work places will not so pointedly demand to know, "What is the pay? How many hours of work per week? Will I get vacation with pay? Is there time and a half for overtime and double time for Sundays?" but instead, or in addition, "What are the harmful exposures incident to this job? How well are these exposures controlled? What is the average work-life expectancy in this trade?"

In this country there are no less than twenty-five thousand different ways to make a living. That was the number widely accepted prior to the exigencies of war; temporarily the number may be even greater. Alphabetically these may range from "accordion makers" to "zooglers"—"zoogler" being the name for the highly skilled balancing artist who rides and steers sawmill logs in soaking ponds up to the hoist. Of these twenty-five thousand or more jobs some three-fourths may involve the use of machines or substances that may be harmful to some or all workers.

"Harm" in this instance is not meant to include the torn flesh, broken bones, damaged eyes, or heat-burned skin that identify the well recognized factory "accidents."

It will be helpful to the ends of this book if at once the cleavage separating industrial accidents from occupational diseases be recognized. The former are instantly or rapidly produced. The crushing of a hand by a punch press, or the dropping of a hammer onto the head of a workman clearly leads to an industrial accident — an accidental injury — a traumatic injury. The nature of these injuries would not have been different if the hand had been crushed at home by a cellar door or the workman's head damaged by a brick falling out of his own chimney. But industry's accidental injuries are not passed over as inconsequential. Moreover, they are far more numerous than the other form of industrial injury soon to be mentioned. In this country, care for victims of unprofitable industrial accidents falls to the lot of industrial physicians, but the prevention and elimination of accidents are within the domain of the safety engineer.

Occupational diseases are caused otherwise. They result from the inimical action of industry's gases, vapors, fumes, mists, solvents, dusts, sensitizers, noises, rays, vibrations, parasites, abnormal atmospheric temperatures and pressures. Such agents do not act instantly; and so the essence of difference between an occupational disease and an accident is the duration of exposure — a little exposure today, a little tomorrow, drop by drop, insidiously brings about an occupational disease. Seemingly, no difficulty should be encountered in defining an occupational disease so that it will not be confused with either the general run of diseases to which all persons are subjected on the one hand or with industrial accidents on the other. To the contrary, one of the traditional courtroom perplexities centers about this rather simple situation. Instead of agreeing that an occupational disease is one caused by exposure at work, most states are guided by the definitional ostentation similar to the one now cited — an illuminating example of the obvious being legally compounded into complexity —

"As used in this act, the term 'occupational disease' means a disease arising out of and in the course of the employment. Ordinary diseases of life to which the general public is exposed outside of the employment shall not be compensable, except where such diseases follow as an incident of an occupational disease as defined in this section. A disease shall be deemed to arise out of the employment, only if there is apparent to the rational mind, upon consideration of all of the circumstances, a direct causal connection between the conditions under which the work is performed and the occupational disease, and which can be seen to have followed as a natural incident of the work as a result of the exposure occasioned by the nature of the employment and which can be fairly traced to the employment as the proximate cause, and which does not come from a hazard to which workmen would have been equally exposed outside of the employment. The disease must be incidental to the character of the business and not independent of the relation of employer and employee. The disease need not have been foreseen or expected but after its contraction, it must appear to have had its origin in a risk connected with the employment and to have flowed from that source as a rational consequence."

All this wordiness merely means—"a disease caused by work."

THE manufacture of the world's goods no longer is a paltry affair. A century ago the textile worker dealt with virgin fibers and few machines, possibly hand looms, and was concerned with a handful of dyes chiefly of vegetable origin. His present day counterpart functions in a welter of detergents, dispersers, leveling agents, mildew preventives, fungicides, finishes, thickening agents, wetters, sizers, desizers, lusters, delusters, softening agents, complex dyes, mordants, toners, lubricants, water repellents, scrooping compounds, humectants, inhibitors, catalysts, and deodorants. It is not denied that all of these innovations lead to products better satisfying or better serving the consumer.

Every other industry has made similar strides. In a single factory recently visited there were found three hundred and forty-three different solvents, oils, and coolants—every one being accepted as having special properties adapted to particular needs. Actually, there was endless, useless duplication.

This fecundity of material innovation is a source of continuous threat to workers in terms of occupational diseases. By no means all, but certainly too many, however serviceable to industry, possess properties inimical to the worker's body or mind.

Concurrently, mighty steps have been taken in warding off these dangers through cunning protective devices. Development in the art of worker protection is never fully abreast of worker dangers. As a consequence, there are this day more occupational diseases than ever before have been recognized by physicians, industrial hygienists, nurses, and dentists.

Through my office pours a cascade of inquiries about occupational diseases, requests for investigations, methods of protection, chemical analyses, expert testimony, all intermingled with patients — some suffering from genuine occupational diseases, some with injuries, many with afflictions which are real enough, but unrelated to work, and a fair number of belligerents. As a rule the degree of belligerency is inversely proportional to the severity or actuality of the disease state.

For the purposes of seeing this domain of medical work, let us dip into this stream an imaginary long-handled net — emulating the dipper of smelts in their hectic upstream rushing.

Our first case is the worker with a severe skin disease involving both lower legs who points out that day by day he stands on a factory floor which has been impregnated with chemicals. He is convinced that in some manner through chemical evaporation an irritation has been brought to his shins. Numerous inquiries are made. A little reluctantly he admits that the week before his difficulty began he bought at high price in black market a dozen pair of the "finest hose." The line of inflammation at the top precisely corresponds with the top of his socks. A small portion of hosiery is snipped off and strapped to his thigh, and within twenty-four hours this brings about a patch of irritation. The diagnosis is obvious. The patient is a little resentful — hatred for himself for having been gullible, hatred for the black market operator who duped him, a dash of hatred for the doctor who knocked the scales off his eyes.

Next comes a letter of inquiry seeking to learn why skin diseases so dominate the occupational disease mosaic. The reply is definite. The worker's nakedness provides his greatest vulnerability. Only the angleworm and his kind are more naked than man. Industry would be better served by a race of men well furred or well feathered, thus interposing a barrier against contact with a myriad of skin irritants. The skin is man's largest organ and one of the most important. It is far from being just a sack into which man is poured. All workers are handicapped by nakedness, but the blondes and redheads harbor additional susceptibility over their brunette and dark-skinned fellows.

A half-conscious truck driver who has sought a little sleep in his cab after an all-night drive is then brought in. The weather is cold and he has elected to let his motor run to provide warmth. The diagnosis may be made instantly—carbon monoxide poisoning. However brainless the accident, it still derives from work. This is an accident, not an occupational disease. The time of exposure was too limited. The employer pays the wholly unnecessary bills.

A request comes to visit Department X, where metal degreasing is done. One by one the workers of the small group have developed nausea, vomiting, and headache as they go about their duties. The degreasers are of the vapor type, and trichlorethylene is the agent that provides the solvent vapors. The machines are well protected. The human element is at fault; the metal being degreased is hoisted in haste without allowing the proper period of drying in the safety zone.

An alarmed secretary presents a dermatitis of her face. In panic she blames the office stationery, the glue on stamps, her carbon paper, her erasers, soap in the washroom. In fact, two days earlier she patronized a beauty parlor to add to her beauty. She secured a permanent. To obtain a hair style pleasing to her vanity a hair lacquer was applied. That chemical contained an irritant. It has done its harm. She is bundled off to her family physician.

Within our day's catch is an old worker. He is short of breath and coughing. Approaching the end of his work days, he is now but a watchman in a car parking lot. An x-ray is made of his chest. There are found the telltale markings of silicosis—a dusty lung disease. He furnishes the story that many years ago, in his prime, he spent twenty years in the stone industry. Slowly the silica dust has produced an incurable disease. It is a physiological miracle that only at his life's twilight has disability come upon him. Removed by two decades from the cause of his disease, the possibility of compensation no longer exists. To him, gently it is suggested that from now on he must let others run the world.

This recital of my day's happenings might be continued without end. But something must be saved for exciting details.

What are the hazardous trades? Almost all trades might have made contributions to this book, and a large number have.

Chapter 3

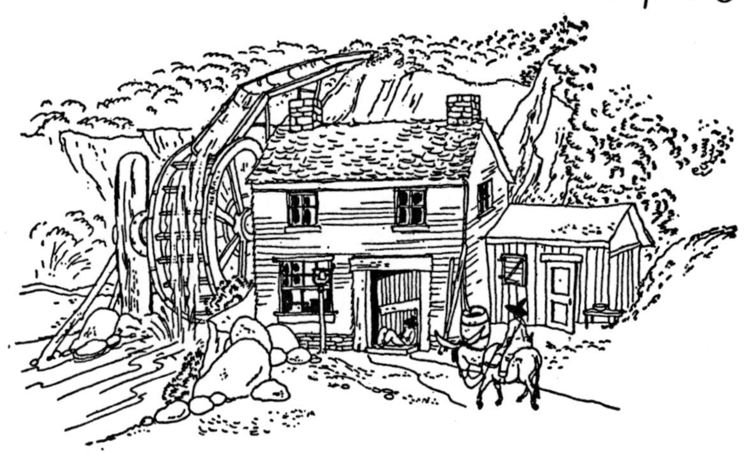

Getting Ready for the Hazardous Trades

HAVING cut my second denture on the granite millstones of neighborhood water-powered grist mills, thus making an acquaintance with dusts; having ridden as my "merry-go-round" the big wooden-cogged, mule-powered wheel that drove primitive cotton gins, thus forming an early kinship with machinery; having warmed my lean toes by the edges of home-made wood tar retorts, contrived by scooping a barrel-sized hole in a clay bank, filling it with pine knots, lighting them with "fat" pine kindling, and allowing the tar to trickle into a wooden pail after flowing along a groove in the hard earth, thus introducing myself to the chemical industry — after all of this it might have been expected that my later appearance at a medical college would have led to my whilly-whally but determined request that I be given opportunity to qualify as an industrial toxicologist or industrial hygienist. I did nothing of the sort. Not having this book in mind at the time, I denied myself a dramatic moment. Had I made the request the inevitable reply would have been, "No medical college in the country would even know about such things."

My choice of a medical college represents a triumph of the nebulous. Working in a Tennessee coal mine in the summer of 1907 and wrestling losingly with the hope that I might get together money enough to go to any medical college, I noted a minor local newspaper item about a medical college at "Ann Harbor." At once there was an irresistible fascination from the possibility of carrying out the gruelling work of the dissecting room and the physiological laboratory where I could relax now and again to view majestic ships plowing through turbulent waters.

Not until the decision was irreversible, did I learn that "Ann Harbor" was "Ann Arbor"—its longest boat possibly a twenty-three foot canoe on the not so large Huron River. Never having seen a steamboat larger than the fist-sized "Nettie Quill" on the Coosa River, my yearning for boats swept me into the University of Michigan captivated by a typographically erring "H."

THE time of birth of a baby is usually a matter of certainty or at least potential certainty—the month, the day, and the hour. The time of birth of a major innovation in medicine usually is and should be unfixable. Try, if you please, to determine the time of the discovery of the microscope so essential to medicine. Some delvers are centuries apart. So it is with the nativity of industrial medicine in America. There is more than a shadow of truth in the unkind observation that some devotees in this field mark its birthday to coincide with the date of their own entry therein. Even in the year of this writing, many "Johnny Come Latelys," climbing onto the outstretched palm of the Titan, promptly begin to shout about "pioneering." This has all the fitness of this month's trail blazing from New York to Philadelphia. Most persons entitled to an opinion would accept either the first or second decade of this century. Desiring the good will of both groups, I make a compromise here, accepting five years of each, thus placing the period of slow birth from 1905 to 1915. Accepting this date is safe enough for me because, reckoned by it, I too am a "Johnny Come Lately."

Long before the beginning of this synthetic decade, there were some noteworthy contributions, but in the twenty-year period between 1880 and 1900 only twenty-two articles were published. Such sparsity fails to reflect any thriving alertness in this field. Much earlier, in 1837, Dr. McCready won a prize offered by the New York State Medical Society for a thesis on "The Influence of Trades, Professions, and Occupations." After a publication drought of thirty-two years, Dr. Walker, of Boston, in 1869 issued a small booklet "Occupations of the People." Ten years later, Dr. Wilson delivered an address on "Diseases Incident to Some Occupations" which was published in the *Transactions of the Medical Society of Youngstown, Ohio,* in 1880. The dearth of published material during this period should serve as a deterrent to some of us who without shame may publish individually as many as twenty-five papers yearly.

In 1885, at the annual meeting of the Public Health Association in Washington, awards were made for four Henry Lomb Prize essays. It is noteworthy that two of the four were concerned with the health of workers. The first of these two prize-winning essays was prepared by Dr. Ireland, of Springfield, Massachussetts, and titled "Preventable Causes of Disease, Injury, and Death in American Manufactories and Workshops." The second, by Dr. Victor Vaughan the elder, of Ann Arbor, was designated "Healthy Homes and Food for the Working Classes." These are the chief published antecedents to the "magnificent decade."

Then came the avalanche. In 1906, by act of the United States Congress the National Committee on Child Labor was created. At about the same time there began a surge of legislative enactments by states relating to compensation for those industrially injured. Some of these laws made provision for occupational diseases. Kober, while serving on one of Theodore Roosevelt's commissions in 1908, submitted to the commission a lengthy report on "Industrial and

Personal Hygiene." Valuable monographs on "The Mortality from Consumption in the Dusty Trades" were contributed by Hoffman in 1908-1909. One year later, the American Association for Labor Legislation sponsored the first National Conference on Industrial Diseases. Again, in 1910, Thompson, a professor of medicine at Cornell University Medical College, brought together an informal committee for appraisal of the significance of occupational diseases in American life. Two years later Alice Hamilton published her pioneering studies of lead poisoning among pottery workers and painters.

This was not all. The National Safety Council was organized in 1911, albeit the health section did not come into being until 1915. The fifteenth International Congress on Hygiene and Dermography held its 1912 sessions in the city of Washington. One of its subdivisions was devoted to the hygiene of occupation. That year, likewise, marked the organization of the American Association of Industrial Physicians and Surgeons, its charter members scarcely more than a score. The textbook, "The Occupational Diseases," by Thompson, one of the truly great creators of occupational disease medicine in this country, first appeared in 1914. In that year Price, of New York, a medical spokesman for labor, published a full length text portraying "The Modern Factory."

The U. S. Public Health Service about 1914 organized a special division of industrial hygiene and sanitation. At the 1914 sessions of the American Public Health Association, Drs. Kober and Hayhurst, both notable in occupational disease work, made addresses that paved the way for a section on industrial hygiene in that association, which section first assembled in New York in 1915. At the time of his address Hayhurst was carrying out his historical survey of occupational diseases in Ohio. About four years earlier Alice Hamilton had completed an Illinois statewide survey of occupational diseases, the first of its scope in America.

This Paricutin-like and never matched decade in the world of industrial medicine was brought to praiseworthy end by the publication of "Diseases of Occupation and Vocational Hygiene," prepared within the "great decade," but not published until 1916. This monument was edited by Dr. George Kober, of Washington, and William C. Hanson, of Belmont, Massachusetts. It is noteworthy that, with two or three exceptions, of the twenty-four American contributors none was well established in the field of occupational diseases, but instead all were workers famous in other fields of medicine who suddenly had been awakened to the importance of occupational diseases in American life.

By the sheerest fortuity, industrial medicine's "great decade" coincides with the decade of my own birth into the world of medicine. Already I was living in a world of industrial hygiene and occupational diseases, but of this I was wholly unaware.

To me as a junior medical student in 1909 came the first clinical touch with occupational diseases.

Dr. Luther Warren, conducting his course in clinical microscopy, blandly stated, "In the clinic tomorrow will be shown a case of lead poisoning. Blood smears are under the microscopes showing stippling in red blood cells. These stipples are diagnostic of lead poisoning."

We know now that that last statement was not factual, but it took some years to prove the contrary. Through a microscope I saw my world for the first time, but I did not then realize that I was viewing at least a symbol of a lifetime of work. No less, there was an undefinable emotional response. This same response was not aroused by other pathological blood cells in specimens from the primary anemias, leukemias, or any other blood dyscrasias. While there was then no world of occupational diseases known to me with which I might form alliance, there was immediately a growing distaste for the lure of surgery, obstetrics, gynecology, or ophthalmology.

For two years more as a student and a few more as a physician I was a "groper" looking for something that existed but of which I didn't know. It took a fire-eating Army colonel—"Two-Gun

Charlie Howland"—to kindle a fire under me. Shortly after the entry of this country into the First World War, and just prior to the influx into a score of camps and cantonments of the nation's draftees, a meager handful of experienced regular Army officers, destined to organize Chicago's "Stockyard Regiment," found themselves surrounded by an eager lot of would-be officers hurriedly trained under make-believe war conditions remote from any firing line. To us, for I was one of them, war at that distance and at that time seemed to be a gentlemen's contest partaking of the qualities of a chess game, skeet shooting, and a picnic on a rainy day. Colonel Howland, then regimental commander but later a general officer, accepted as one of his chief functions the "toughening up" of his officers in order that the stark brutality of actual war might be sensed and accepted. His language, always picturesque, was not always printable. In exasperation he thundered at his puerile lot of prospective regimental officers, "Men, when you get into battle you will find yourself and your men about you mercilessly sticking bayonets into the bellies of your enemy and, in your excitement to get on to the next oncoming enemy, twirling out the guts of your foe. That is warfare, and when you have once done that, you'll never shoot ducks again."

Turning to me, as the newly appointed regimental surgeon, he sarcastically added, "We have here an experimental physiologist, who has spent years with a hundred thousand tadpoles, trying to figure out what changes them into frogs. When he gets into battle and has lying around him within his own responsibility one hundred men with jaws shot off, crushed chests, gouged-out eyes, bullet wounds through the liver, he is going to realize that working with men, not with tadpoles, is the real game."

That flailing marked the turning of a youthful research physiologist away from tadpoles, mice, and guinea pigs to bigger game, human beings, and to a particular set of human beings, industrial workers, and a particular set of diseases, the diseases of industrial workers. First though, there was a war to be won.

Favoring fortune later caused me to be stationed as the Chief of Laboratory Services in an Army camp where there served as the chief of another service, Christian R. Holmes, in civilian life the Dean of the Medical College of the University of Cincinnati. One happy morning shortly after the Armistice Colonel Holmes announced that he was more needed as a dean than as an Army officer and that he was leaving. Anyone knowing this officer might well believe that it would scarcely occur to him to arrange for a formal discharge or patiently await an Army order relieving him from his duties. More likely he merely sent a fatherly telegram to his friend, the Secretary of War, called his car, stowed his duffel, and casually instructed some assistant to procure his discharge. Exactly what this greatly loved, but little conforming temporary Army officer did, is not known. At any rate, he left. That war was over.

Before leaving he came to me, not with a question or a request but with a surprising statement: "Major, you will be needed here in the Army a little longer. Get your discharge when you can and then come to me. You are going to head up a new School of Public Health in our university, which you and I are going to build."

"But," I protested, "I know little about public health in general—only a few high spots. I know nothing about public health administration, and that is probably your greatest need."

The departing officer waved his hand in deprecation and said, "Never mind. I have seen you in action for the past eighteen months. What you don't possess we will find in somebody else. For years you have wanted to investigate workers' diseases. Here is your opportunity. Come on to me."

I did join that medical officer, now restored to his deanship, but with trepidation. That was May of 1919. No formal arrangements were made. In my lifetime thus far I have found four men who stirred in me a full willingness to follow blindly, to ask no questions, to anticipate nothing save fairness and opportunity. The dean was one of those four. His instructions on my arrival were not detailed, but they were adequate: "Spend the summer here. Meet the people of this city. Meet the faculty. Decide what you and I must do in order to make the beginnings of the best public health school in America. I am going away now on a trip to the Arctic Ocean. In the fall we will really get under way. By that time have a plan and a good one. You will find moneys available for your summer's needs at the treasurer's office. I have arranged for that."

The good dean went away. He did not return alive.

His death was a blow to a school, a city, a state and the nation — for me, disaster. Only a few weeks earlier I had burned my bridges to the past, and now the bridges to the future were burned even before their building. I found myself on a tiny atoll, but at least I was free, free to move in any direction. At least so I thought, but really there was no choice; there was always the "ding, ding" toward the worker, his hurts, occupational diseases, industrial hygiene. Industrial hygiene, now on the lips of every person, then as a division of public health scarcely was freed of its vernix caseosa. (Here I find myself dropping into the language of the doctor, which for the purposes of this book I have foresworn.) If you be concerned to know what "vernix caseosa" is, let it be described as nature's lubricant at the time of birth.

In the midst of much self-goading, and of more goading by the remembered scorn of the old Colonel, I was well aware that I was painfully handicapped. I knew nothing about industrial hygiene or occupational diseases. I had never been in large numbers of factories. My knowledge of workers was scant. These shortcomings were known to others, and they indulged in the lifted eyebrow and tongue in cheek. In part I was shoved, not rocked, into industrial hygiene. Having never been in factories, I had to learn about them. If there was experience to be gained, I would gain it; if there were few known occupational diseases, I would find more. I determined to have a share in the world of workers.

To the way of thinking of many physicians, professionally one may be in only four places — at the bedside, in the consultation room, in the hospital, at the academy of medicine. With a fair degree of tolerance these physicians accept the insurance doctor, the ship's physician, the medical public health officer, the medical teacher and the military surgeon, but rarely are they taken to the profession's bosom. Their enterprises are regarded as rather unfortunate happenings, though not entirely deplorable. In early days, more of ire than tolerance was held for physicians who aligned themselves with industry for the purposes of the protection of the health of workers and who called themselves "industrial physicians." Privately such physicians were sometimes labeled "renegades," "degenerates." For use in public there was created the disapprobative term "contract physician." This term had a little nastiness in it and could be used in public with just the proper inflection to indicate that much more might be said on the subject did not courtesy intervene. In those days to enter the field of industrial health conservation carried with it the penalty of being shorn of a few of the outer garments of medical respectability.

To a few of us, however, there was given the boon of prescience — the foresight of the country's tremendous industrial expansion, the concurrent rise in occupational diseases. So girdled, the sneering of the majority was not minded. The zealot never minds.

In 1919 industrial medicine was no "Field of the Cloth of Gold." It was a field of anathema. Quite without any martyrdom, I gaily accepted the badge of professional degradation. In 1919 I became an industrial physician.

IN RETROSPECT, the lack of knowledge of trade diseases at that period was appalling. My own ignorance was teeming. In this present day, when every school child beyond the fifth grade may speak knowingly about radium poisoning or the nature of "diver's" disease, it has become well-nigh unbelievable that only twenty-five years ago few physicians could have even named more than five occupational diseases and that — more distressing to confess — half of the little we thought we knew had no basis in fact. Silicosis, the king of the occupational diseases, now known to be solely the result of chemical action, was then attributed to the cutting of the lungs by sharp-edged sand particles, much like the action that takes place in the grinding up of food in a chicken's gizzard.

Some of us discoursed stupidly, but as we thought learnedly, about muscular cramps in workers caused by the drinking of highly cold water. I have written well-meant gems on the subject, perhaps drinking well chilled water the while and not having cramps and not questioning the lack of evidence within my own body. We now know that workers' cramps on hot days are due to the loss from the body of ordinary salt in the process of sweating.

My particular contribution to futility was long months spent in an effort to put on a substantial basis a non-existent disease — chronic carbon monoxide poisoning. Ever since man's first discovery of fire the commonest physiologic deviation of the human body has been caused by carbon monoxide gas but always as an acute affair. From the very nature of the action of carbon monoxide no chronic poisoning may arise. The prospects of my having made a contribution were not better than the prospect of a long life for an ice cream cone in an orphans' home. What our small group of pioneers lacked in facts was thoroughly concealed by fervor. But be not disarmed by all the glorification of the marvels of the present; we industrial hygienists still are wonderfully ignorant.

It is fortunate that in those early years there was no immediate and widespread demand for my services, since I had no real services to offer. The laboratory instruments making up my physical equipment were a sling psychrometer for measuring humidity, a foot-candle meter to test factory illumination, and a primitive form of dust counter. Appraised by standards of today the accuracy of that dust counter could not have been greater than ten per cent. Unaware of its shortcomings, I fondled it as a symbol of the magnificent investigations that lay somewhere ahead. Having little entree to industry, I made dust counts of the air in streets, in trolley cars, in churches. No one paid a great deal of attention to me, but I was getting ready for a lifetime of work in the hazardous trades.

The mental equipment that must be ever ready for immediate use by the average practitioner of medicine is enormous, but that which must be possessed by the physician in industry is prodigious. Starting at least on a parity with the practitioner, he in addition must know much about occupational diseases and industrial hygiene. Then comes his greatest need — familiarity with industry itself, its machines, materials, language, products, by-products, waste products. In a single factory it is not extraordinary to find as many as two hundred different types of machines, each performing a different task and perhaps utilizing somewhat different adjuvants such as cutting oils, water-soluble oils, soda water, quenching oils, pickling wash, brighteners, antioxidants. Every trade and often an individual plant has its own language. In a given plant a certain part, to the planning and operating committee, might be known as 469D-TY8122; throughout the plant this same part might be known as the "turtle back."

Nearly all of industry is amazingly complex. Casting about for some industry intimate to our persons and likely to be regarded as simple, let us take button manufacture. In the first place there are shell buttons, metal buttons, fabric buttons, bone buttons, glass buttons, plastic buttons, wooden buttons, rubber buttons and leather buttons. For all classes the operations are highly different and numerous.

Any similarity between the processes devoted to the manufacture respectively of pearl buttons and plastic buttons may be limited to the fact that both begin with "B." Operations on a pearl button start with the collection of mussels from some river such as the Mississippi. The manufacture of plastic buttons starts with some chemical constituent such as phenol. A worker in a pearl button mill desiring to transfer his skill to the plastic button industry would find himself as unfamiliar with plastic procedures as with processes in the manufacture of parts for a gyro compass. In the aggregate of all of its branches, button manufacture entails no less than five hundred distinct work steps.

Laying aside the stethoscope and the thermometer, the industrial physician, if truly he is to qualify in this unusual field of medical work, must know the details of tens of thousands of operations — even button manufacture. I learned much detail and, if proof is required, I refer to my publication on pearl buttons made long ago and deeply buried, but, for a little-changing industry, I hope still accurate.

So near at hand a device as the storage battery in your automobile involved no less than four hundred dissimilar operations before it could have been sold to you as workable. For an entire automobile the number approximates thirty thousand. A brake pedal alone, not including the rubber cushion slipped over it, requires under the most economical number of manufacturing stages thirty-two separate operations.

In the lean years, waiting for clients, I sought to become familiar with the manufacture of all wares from thimbles to tractors, from school crayons to locomotives, from fish hooks to machine guns, from toothpastes to steel girders. At one time with glibness I might have named the two hundred and four industries then using lead in some form. Every day for five years I carried on my person a laboriously compiled code which at a glance told me the commoner threats to workers in more than two thousand trades. I was becoming an industrial hygienist, but at first only a rocking-chair industrial hygienist.

Biding time was not too onerous, for with good eyesight I saw ahead tall adventures, adventures in miniature, adventures underground in mines, overhead in planes, in books, in homes, in factories, in court rooms, in legislative halls, but, very especially, adventures in the hearts of people. Getting ready for these adventures was in itself an adventure, but for many months after I seemed to be ready the most important thing in all of living was the coming of the first job. For this I waited.

One fine day the first job did come. I had no warning. A long distance telephone call from another state allowed no time for conferences, no time to think. I was invited to carry out an investigation of an unknown occupational disease under emergency circumstances. The telephone caller introduced himself as "Mr. Fiferlik," the manager of a railway crosstie treating plant for one of the country's great trunk lines. He explained, "About half of my men have a bad skin disease. Some of them are so bad it looks like cancer to me. Unless I can give them some promise today, they're going to walk out on me. What'll I tell them?"

I was frightened, too. I didn't know what he should tell them. Despite my long months of preparation and efforts to anticipate every contingency, here was the long awaited first job in an industry of which I had never heard. Mustering a lot of boldness that I really didn't possess, I shouted, evenly I hope, "Just tell them I'll be there tomorrow morning and that in a few days this trouble will be in hand." He was relieved. Over the telephone rolled the burden — from his shoulders to mine.

As I put down the receiver, my secretary inquired, a little weakly, "Now what are you going to do?" Quite honestly, I answered, "I don't know."

But here is the story of the first job; and then came others, for in the ensuing years there have been many hundreds.

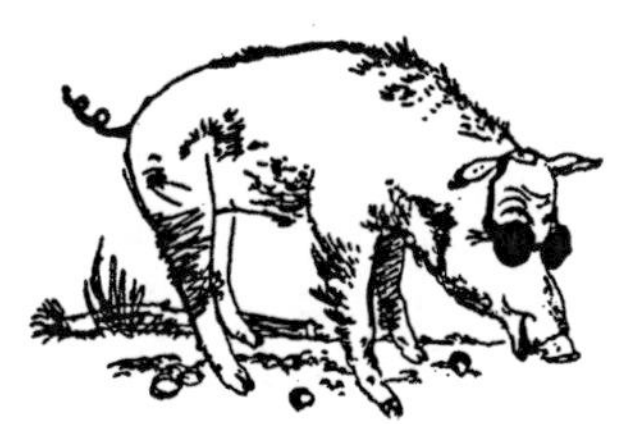

Chapter 4

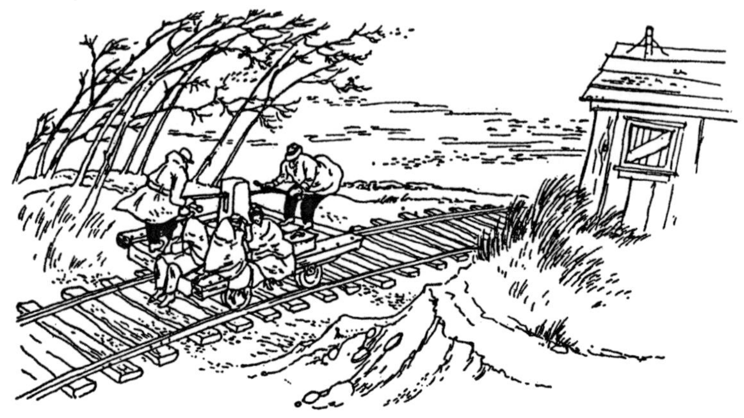

The First Job

I was launched into my career as an industrial hygienist on a handcar. How fortunate this was, for twenty-five years later, even as I write about it, that handcar challenges interest. Had I gone by pullman to my first job, no one, perhaps, would now be willing to accompany me further along this stream of betidings.

From the moment of the telephone call and until our departure next morning, we made hurried preparations. Long before this event we had made arrangements with Mrs. Margaret Gilman to serve as the laboratory's staff photographer when the need arose and had similarly established rapport with a chemistry instructor at the University of Cincinnati. Fortunately both were available for the first journey. Augmented by a secretary, we were a staff of four. Surrounded now for the first time by a staff, may I not introduce some "we's" among the "I's"?

According to plan, we met at the station and departed in train No. 86 at seven A.M. with the mercury well near zero. Hours later at a station known as Benson we were greeted by an apologetic plant manager and a slight surprise. The tie treating plant, we learned, was in no town, and because of mountains it was then accessible only by railroad. The nearest passenger stop, Benson, was twenty miles distant, and freight trains paused at the plant only to drop carload lots of untreated ties or to pick them up after treatment. While arrangements might be made to stop any passenger or freight trains on one or two occasions, our daily transportation requirements would be out of the question. In shivering impatience we listened out his preface, which left us none the less unprepared for the denouement. With bluish fingers he pointed to a handcar, remarking that his chief concern was for the ladies. He hadn't counted on the ladies, and we hadn't counted on the handcar. Despite his thoughtful provision of a blanket for each one of us, our chattering teeth and the noise of the car made conversation en route impossible.

But there was time for thinking. For the moment I began to doubt the values of charting the unexplored world of occupational diseases and to envy the lot of the pediatrists who go about their duties in the extra warmth of nurseries and cradles. Then I recalled some of the things that babies do and promptly realigned myself with occupational diseases. At least they occur only in adults. In my half-frozen state there came the recollection of my very first job as a boy.

At the age of twelve I became the sexton of a church at the satisfactory salary of $1.00 monthly. This was not the first dollar I had earned. Within the family, I had been voted a dollar for complete reading of the New Testament. This represents the greatest quantity of energy I have ever expended in the earning of a single dollar. As a sexton my duties were numerous and my responsibilities great. I filled the many lamps with kerosene, trimmed the wicks, and cleaned the glass chimneys, swept the church, dusted the altar, built fires in the stoves and and stacked up hymnals. The most pleasant part was ringing the church bell precisely on time: first and second bell; bells for Sunday school; then for the morning church service;

for the meeting of the "Sunbeams" in the Sunday afternoon; two rings for the night service. This was repeated for the Wednesday evening prayer meeting. The worst times were the periods of protracted meetings — every day and night for two weeks in a row. At least there were no fires to be kindled during the summer protracted meetings and services; but there was no extra pay for these extra duties. All of that job was clear-cut, definite.

Now nothing was definite. "Now," I queried myself, "just what is ahead of me ten miles down this track?" I comforted myself with the old adage, "Nothing is truly hard when you get to it."

A half hour later, well covered with snow, we arrived at the crosstie plant. In a warm office, the manager described the work operations and later his woes. Untreated crossties were brought in from various points in flat car lots. After due weathering for drying, batches of these ties were loaded on trams and moved into huge cylinders, sealed off, and flooded with a hot mixture of tar and zinc chloride under pressure. The zinc chloride was introduced for fire prevention and to repel the action of rot-producing bacteria and fungi, while the tar was applied as a waterproofing agent. To increase the fluidity of the tar heat was required, and pressure was utilized to force the chemical mixture deeply into the woody interstices. Following treatment, the dripping ties were stacked in piles in the plant area; this was in part a hand operation.

The procedure had been carried on for several years without difficulty until two weeks previously when a few of the men had developed a blistering rash on the forearms and the backs of the hands. Soon more workers were affected. The rash spread to shoulders, chest, and neck regions, and several workers reported involvement of knees and thighs. In one group deep ulcers developed along with infection.

Little work was being performed. The plant was in a panic, threatened with a complete work stoppage. Fiferlik indicated that unless prompt action be started it might be necessary to close the plant at the end of that day, but it was also his opinion that our

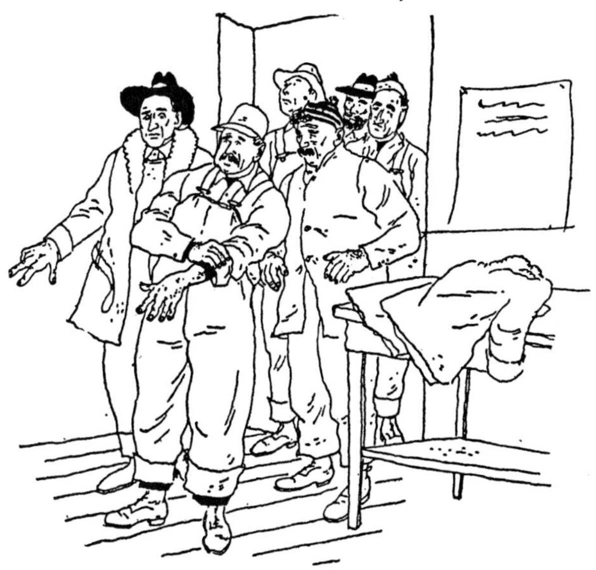

presence would go far toward allaying apprehension among the workers.

Thus informed, I suggested that several of the men, the leaders among the disturbers, be called in for some reassurance. In walked a dozen tarry, begrimed laborers, eager to express their dreads and exhibit their injured skins, but anxious to continue their work if safe. I told them frankly that we did not know the exact cause of the troublesome skin disease, but that no common skin disease from work, however discomforting and painful, was likely to threaten life or persist for any great length of time. They were assured that every man would be examined and supplied with some soothing palliative remedy, while action to discover the source of irritation would promptly be started. The chemist was pointed out as competent to investigate any injurious constituents; and shortly he was examining every operation on the premises, collecting his samples. In a makeshift examining room, I began to look over the afflicted workers one by one, asking for them in the order of their severity. The photographer was on hand to take pictures of damaged hands, arms and knees, while the secretary recorded my findings.

It was obvious that the dermatitis was chemical in origin and not an infection that might be attributed to bacteria, yeasts or fungi. A shipment of a mild ointment known to be efficacious in almost all varieties of chemical dermatitis was ordered from the city by long distance telephone, and the first day of the first job ended.

Since tar cancer, as represented by "chimney sweep cancer," was one of the earliest recognized occupational diseases, it was conceived as possible that one or two cases of low grade skin cancer actually might exist. Of this we were never quite certain.

"The hell of it all," the manager would mutter in profound perplexity, "the hell of it is that we've been doing these same operations identically, month in month out, year after year, without anything like this happening before."

Exactly that was disturbing to us too. The enigma was not that the skin disease was widespread, but that after years of exposure, an explosive outbreak should appear.

"Same operations — year after year — never happened before," this pounded through my brain all day and became the broken record of my sleep at night. Days went by, every one bringing scattered shreds of new information. When the weather was good, we were able to get to the plant by automobile over a semblance of a road. On bad days we leaned on the handcar, depending on the train dispatcher at Benson for the right of way. Infrequently, we traveled in the caboose of the occasional freight train that stopped. With no thought of paying fares, we reached the high estate of hoboes. Only two trips were made by the photographer. Her duties were finished. The secretary, a good campaigner, hung on longer, but eventually only the chemist and I, day by day, lived the life of the crosstie treater.

"Year in year out — the same operations — never trouble before." Why? A tiny, single fact proved to be the key. With chagrin we realized that we had not made adequate inquiry sooner. Just before the epidemic a new shipment of tar had been received, routine fulfillment of a routine order. It seemed the hottest clew of the pursuit thus far. Taking several of the workmen known to be sensitive to the chemicals, we exposed portions of their right forearms to bits of tar culled from one of the old shipment vats. No less anxiously than the workmen actively involved did we wait for the result of the test, and with no less satisfaction did we observe the final outcome — no trace of irritation. Simultaneously the left forearms had been exposed to minute applications of tar from the new shipment, and almost immediately inflammation occurred. The cause of the skin disease was rapidly unfolding. Although purporting to be the same and sold on identical specifications, the new lot actually was a different type of tar.

Preventive means were now obvious. "Get rid of the offending tar and get no more like it." We were a little ashamed that we had not spotted the trouble-maker earlier. Twenty-five years later, with hundreds of similar episodes behind us, almost our first inquiry would have been about "new shipments"— but that was our first job.

After a few days no new cases appeared. No strike and no threats of strikes. We provided better gloves, aprons, washing facilities. The friendly workers held up unscarred, undamaged arms. Always it was, "Look, doctor, I am all well now." The epidemic dissolved into nothingness.

Once or twice every year, travel takes me past this isolated industrial plant. So far as I know no other occupational disease outbreak ever has occurred. Whenever I see that plant from a train window, a low bow is made to the beginning of some twenty-four hundred other studies, large and small, completed during the ensuing twenty-five years.

Most of all I remember that I was launched into my career as an industrial hygienist on a railroad handcar.

Another kind of handcar, the type pushed around in factories, shoved Hannah, the laundry worker, against a steam pipe. This handcar changed Hannah's history for a time and provides warrant for linking her oncoming story with my own.

Chapter 5

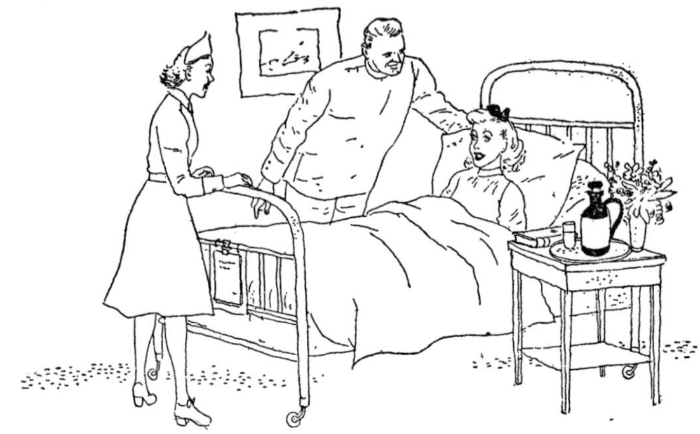

Hannah's Hand

HAVING broken the ice with our first job, other items of investigative work rapidly came to our doors. One of these was a request from the State's Industrial Accident Board to act as a consulting referee or investigator for disputed occupational disease or unusual injury claims. Out of this connection, which lasted for many years, came acquaintance with Hannah.

The beginning of this adventure was a cryptic letter from the Board which, in part, read:

Re: Hannah MacMuircertais
Y-17812089

Dear Doctor:

In the town of Ogden, near your own city, Dr. John Pharis, with offices at 89 Walnut Street, has had under his care for nearly two years the above captioned claimant. This Board is of the opinion that this claimant's condition should be more thoroughly investigated, which opinion is shared by Dr. Pharis, who himself has requested some assistance. This doctor has been notified of your appointment as the special investigator in this case.

> We are especially concerned to have any information that may account for the prolongation of what was apparently only a moderately severe injury. We do not wish to make further statements at this time in order that we may not hamper you in your own inquiries. Will you please make arrangements with Dr. Pharis and in time make appropriate report to this office?

The next day in Ogden Dr. Pharis gave every evidence of being willing to share a disagreeable responsibility with another physician. Perplexity hung heavily in the atmosphere of his office.

"This case," he said by way of introduction, "is either the most amazing I have ever had in my surgical practice, or else I am a sorry specimen of a surgeon."

He drew a sheaf of progress charts from his drawer, and noting their thickness I settled back in my chair. Hannah's history followed.

"This girl," Dr. Pharis began, "is now twenty years old. When she was seventeen, she began working in the local laundry, on the mangle I believe, and had to take out working papers on this account. One day, when she had been working about a year, she was passing through a narrow aisle in the laundry and was somehow pinned against a steam pipe, by a handcar, with her hand caught behind her. The back of the hand was pressed against the hot pipe for some seconds. I was called in and took the girl into the city to the Farnsworth Hospital. She was badly frightened by the accident and further upset by the hospital, never having been in one before. After a time, however, she became quite accustomed to the new routine and adjusted herself remarkably. She was the model patient, knew the nurses and interns by name, and was popular among the ward patients.

"At the proper time," Dr. Pharis continued, "I carried out a skin graft for Hannah's hand, using a pedicle graft from her thigh. The result was beautiful, one of my very best. Three weeks later she left the hospital, loaded down with gifts, and returned home. By arrangement, she reported to my office every third day — for observation rather than treatment — until, a few weeks later, I decided she could return to work. That would have been the next Monday following a Thursday examination.

"That Saturday she came into the office highly agitated, tears running down her cheeks. The hand was wrapped in an improvised bandage. She rushed in to me saying 'Look! Look!' and I found that the entire graft had been destroyed by deep ulceration. There was no indication of infection, but the area was violently inflamed.

"I can tell you," Pharis said, throwing the charts down on the desk, "that came as something of a shock. Her progress to that point had been normal and most satisfactory. I had heard about auto-sensitization in skin grafts and had long wanted to see it, but hardly in one of my own patients."

"Did she have any explanation?" I asked.

"No, none. She said that during the previous afternoon her hand had become swollen and painful with a few small ulcerations here and there over the grafted area. Her sleep had been fitful, and the hand had given her pain throughout the night; however, she paid little attention to it until morning, when she found it as she showed it to me."

"Odd," I remarked.

"For my own explanation," he resumed, "I merely told her that as healing takes place certain chemical changes occur in the proteins, and that on rare occasions the proteins themselves may act as poison. Obviously she had to go back to the hospital, and she accepted the fact quite stoically. We put her in the same wing with the same friends, and made everything as pleasant as possible for her. She had a new story to tell about the 'allergic' loss of her skin graft."

Dr. Pharis thumbed through the charts again and picked up the story. "I was able to carry out another skin graft using a flap from the other thigh. In spite of the scarring related to the previous ulceration we again obtained a good graft. Her recovery was complete. However, having experienced the loss of one graft through some bizarre allergy, I kept Hannah in the hospital two weeks longer. After she had been a short period at home and at a time when the hand was in excellent condition, I again told her she could resume her duties at the laundry, whereupon we lost the second graft. It all happened in much the same manner as the first, and the process was repeated yet a third time. She now has her fourth graft, which naturally isn't as good as the first because of so much surgical interference. Right now is the time that she's due to lose it if she runs true to the other three. I've read everything available on the auto-digestion of grafted materials, but nothing really fits this." He shook his head in mute exasperation.

We were silent for a time. "Tell me something more about Hannah herself," I urged. "What has her background been?"

"Usual, or perhaps a little worse than usual — low family, poverty, shabbiness."

"She lives alone," I mused.

"Her mother died a year ago, I believe." Pharis' voice was tired.

"And she got along well at the hospital?"

"It was a new world for her," Dr. Pharis exclaimed. "She almost seemed to enjoy it — food with silver service, nurses bathing her, changing her linen, combing her hair. Why shouldn't she get along well?" The office nurse interrupted us at that moment. "Miss MacMuircertais is here," she informed us.

Pharis turned to me questioningly. "Let's talk to her," I decided.

Hannah entered, a small red-headed girl with eyes that moved constantly. She appeared slightly nervous, ill at ease in the presence of two doctors. I was introduced as a visiting surgeon; and Hannah was invited to tell her own story, which she did with considerable facility. Having had months of contact with surgeons and nurses, Hannah knew all of the terms — "third degree burns," "necrosis," "pedicle grafts," "autolysis," "sensitization," "allergy," "drainage." The recital was merely a repetition of what Dr. Pharis had previously told me.

"And when," Hannah finished, "when do you think I can go back to work?" She looked from one to the other of us and dropped her eyes to her hands, folded in her lap.

"You will be quite ready to return next Monday, barring accident," her doctor announced. I nodded agreement. Hannah smiled.

"Just one suggestion," I offered. "Suppose we use some solution on the hand that will toughen the skin against the eventuality of further harm at the laundry." Dr. Pharis looked surprised, as well he might, but I continued hastily. "Miss MacMuircertais, if you will return at this time tomorrow, we'll apply this toughening medicament."

Hannah agreed and left immediately.

"It occurs to me," I told the puzzled Pharis, "that Hannah isn't allergic to anything but her environment."

"You think she's destroying her own grafts?" he exclaimed.

That was exactly my suspicion. Before the next afternoon we obtained a solution of thymolphthalein, a water-like fluid without irritant properties. Hannah arrived promptly, and we instructed her in the application of the solution. First we applied a few turns of bandage around the hand, not enough to hide all of the skin graft, and advised her to keep this wrapping wet with small quantities of the solution furnished her. She was given extra bandage and told that if the original binding became soiled she might apply fresh bandage. By this time she had become quite proficient in bandaging her own injury.

It was anticipated that if Hannah were to lose her fourth skin graft the event probably would take place within the next two days, since she was scheduled to return to work four days later. Dr Pharis made out his final papers, certified the girl for work, praised her for being the perfect patient, and told her she need not return unless something unusual happened.

The following day, Friday, the unusual, if not the unexpected, did happen. I was waiting in Dr. Pharis' office when Hannah was announced by the nurse. She came in looking startled and worried, innocently exhibiting the hand. Her bandage and her skin were a brilliant sky blue. Over the grafted surface were a few minor ulcerations, also blue.

"Doctor," she said in a low voice, "I think I'm losing this graft too, but it's not starting like the others. I never saw this blue color before." She was frightened.

"Sit down, Hannah," I said, and I hope triumph was not in my voice. "I want you to hear a story."

She obeyed automatically, still staring at the hand.

"The story is about a girl who worked in a laundry. This girl wasn't very old, but she had worked hard throughout her life. The work in the laundry was hard and the pay not very high, but the girl didn't mind because in her whole lifetime everything that she had done was hard. She had no family to go home to after work, and the room in which she lived was shabby and lonely, always filled with the outside noises of other people's children. Then one day this girl who worked in a laundry got her hand burned rather badly. It was necessary for her to stay in the hospital for many weeks. There everything was spotlessly clean, and nicer things, perhaps even nicer people, than the girl had ever known were an everyday part of life. The doctors and nurses were all happy, even some of the patients were happy, and this girl was the center of much interest. Doctors came and went; nurses were at her beck and call. It was only necessary to press a button at the head of the bed and almost anything she wanted was hers. For the first time in her life she was important."

Hannah was staring at me, wide-eyed.

"Then," I continued, "the time came for this girl to return to her own home, her room. Her good doctor had saved her hand, and she could go back to work. There would be no more compensation benefits from her employer's insurance company, but she could work for herself again. At home, however, the girl found she was lonesome for her friends the nurses, the interns, the surgeons, the orderlies, the waitresses. She had to cook her own food, wash her own dishes, mend her own clothes, comb her own hair; and she was alone, always alone. The thought of the laundry was unbearable — heat, steam, odors, noises."

The small face before me was white and strained.

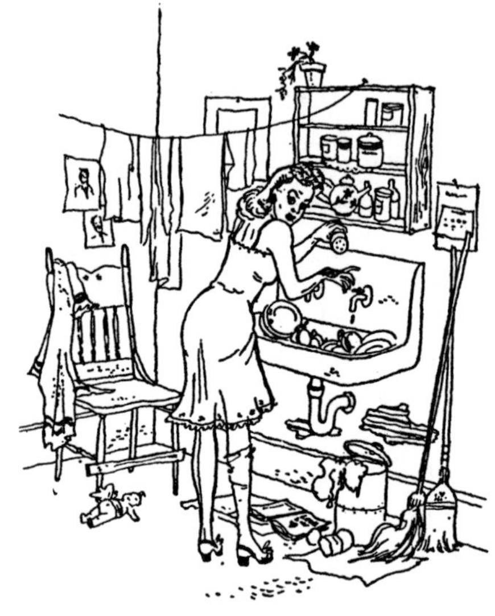

"So this girl sought to escape the necessity of returning to the old life. Over her sink was a can of lye used to clean out a stopped-up drain pipe. It was labeled 'Poisonous — Caustic.' No less, this lonesome girl wetted her hand a little and then put flakes of lye on the surface of her skin graft. Surprisingly it didn't hurt. You see skin grafts have no nerve supply until a long time after the graft is applied."

Hannah was sobbing in frightened despair. "What are you going to do with me? Why is my hand all blue?"

"Hannah, you are, of course, the girl I have been talking about. The white medicine that we gave you always turns a vivid blue when any strong alkali is brought in contact with it. We suspected you were burning off your grafts, but this one is going to be all right. You lost your nerve when you saw the blue color and washed away most of the lye. These little burns will get well promptly."

"What are you going to do?" she begged me. "Will they put me in jail? Will I have to pay back all that money?" There was no defiance in her attitude, merely abject fright.

Dr. Pharis, whose trust had been so abused, became the defiant one on hearing the story later; but we decided Hannah would not be prosecuted.

"No, Hannah, we will make a little bargain. If you will go on back to work, much as you dislike it — if you will put up with your home, bad as it is for a while, we'll keep your secret from all but a very few people."

So, when you pass through the laundry, if you see a young and pretty red-head with a skin graft on the back of her hand, about three inches square, you mustn't give the secret away. That may be Hannah.

THWARTING a foolish, attention-loving Hannah warranted no pride in achievement save possibly from having saved her from her silly self. Far from rating our maneuver as despicable, the members of the Accident Board, furnished with precise proof of a long perpetuated raid on semi-public funds, were so loud in their praise that we gratefully but secretly rated them as our publicity department. Soon we were engulfed in a work world of gases, vapors, dusts and skin irritants, involving cases and consultations, conferences, claims, hearings, lawsuits and trials. Since dust long has been the presiding devil over the evil sources of occupational diseases, there is reason aplenty here to give a dusty flavor to the next four of the adventures that make up this book.

Chapter 6

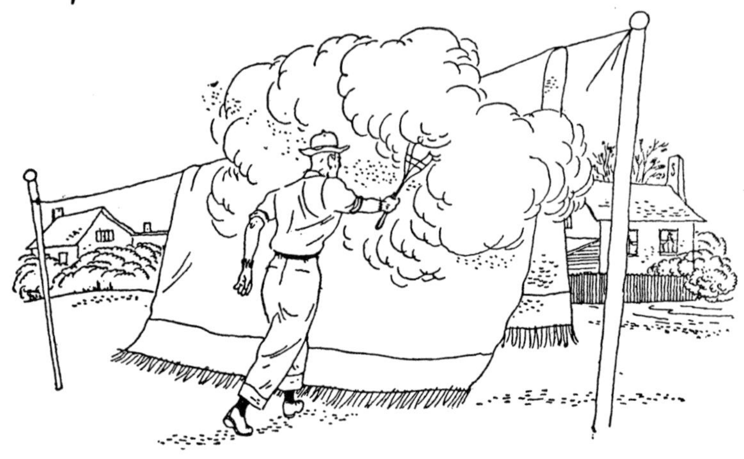

Dust is a Friend and a Foe

MAN lives on the terrasphere surrounded by the atmosphere; fish inhabit the aquasphere; birds chiefly frequent the arborasphere; planes reach the stratosphere; but industrial hygienists in particular deal with the konisphere — the world of dust. Since there is a tacit agreement temporarily to share the tasks of one industrial hygienist, it becomes desirable to step into his aura of dust.

Already you live in your own aura of dust and have from your first breath of life. Your last breath of life, like your first, will contain dust. You thus are making no new acquaintance. Not one cubic foot of air on earth is wholly free of dust. Seeking the best of natural air for your breathing, still you would daily take into your body some two hundred million particles of dust. Dust is one of the earth's magnificent commonplaces. Go, as you have done, into a darkened room which has just one aperture — a knot hole or a crevice — through which brilliant sunshine streams. Enough dust may be seen at a glance to furnish proof of much that this recital would have you share.

Dust is a friend. Without it no clouds, no rain, no snow, no colorful sunsets. Among other needs for this old world — this one huge dust heap — is that about once every ten years there shall be a volcanic eruption on a grand scale. Volcanoes are the artists that make the sunsets later painted by lesser artists. If you are disturbed over the volcanic eruption, a full-sized forest fire will do the trick. Don't worry over the distribution. A first class eruption in Guatemala may furnish food for the poet's pen in Ireland. A forest fire in Oregon may add brilliance to sunsets in Spain. If your interest in dust be merely local and money minded, then buy your farm ten or twenty miles downwind from a cement factory. Enough alkali dust will be deposited to slake the thirst of any alkali-hungry crop.

Quit using the thoroughly eroded and erring figure of speech 'pure as snow.' Snow flakes never would have formed except for the impurity of dust. Every flake contains at least one mote of dust.

When the dusky behemoth who in theory stands between me and dust on my furniture, muttered at the verge of profanity about the endless dust through the "winders," I protested in raillery, "Josie, shame on you. You should be a dust worshiper and address it in adoration, 'O, Thou, Mighty Protector.' Daily it saves your life. In fact without dust you never would have been born, because everybody would have been dead before you."

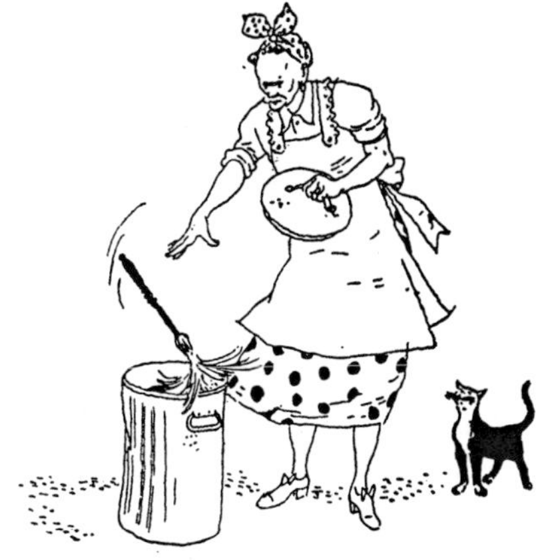

"How tell, Doctor?" inquired Josie.

I, always looking for an audience, did tell. "You see, Josie, all clouds are built around dust. These clouds hold back deadly rays from the sun. If they ever get through, exit Josie; exit Doctor. Throughout the world there have been sun worshipers, moon worshipers, fire worshipers, grain worshipers. Only because man's friend 'dust' in its most helpful forms is invisible has the world escaped a dust-worshiping cult."

Josie in turn — a little uncertain that she wasn't being ribbed — gasped, "Doctor, if all you says is true, I ain't ever goin' to disturb dust no more."

That pedantry boomeranged. Now that dust is sacred, I have more dust. Notwithstanding, up to this point I have been friendly to dusts. Most dusts are friendly, but have few friends.

But dust is also a foe — some dust. Most bad dusts are merely pestiferous, some are temporarily discomfiting, a few are mortal enemies. My one time small daughter in tribute to the odors of hollyhocks was wont to stick her not too aquiline nose into the flower cup. The enemy in the form of pollen dust immediately set about the business of temporarily producing a bulbous nose that might compete with any of the rhinosclerotic noses of the back alley besodden.

Of the first-flight dust foes — there are not so many — lead, mercury, arsenic, manganese, fluorides, etc., silica is the archfiend. Among occupational diseases, silicosis (the lung disease produced by fine silica) is the grave-digger. The history of labor is pockmarked with records of silicosis under some name such as "potter's rot," "miner's asthma," "stone hewer's phthisis," "dust consumption."

Tragedy from silicosis at Gauley Bridge, West Virginia, a catastrophe within the time even of those now in high schools, is the real but little recognized national disgrace from which stems much of the current feverish surge of industrial worker protection. In the midst of a hurried-up hydroelectric tunnelling operation men died by the hundreds. All were grossly exposed to silica dust with but the semblance of protection. That is not my story. I cannot record the sorry details.

Some fifteen thousand other workers in dusty trades in twenty-two states have passed through the mills of medical examination within my charge — dust counts, chemical analyses, x-rays of chests, x-rays of dusts, disability ratings, autopsies, incineration of lung samples. Some have proved hale and hearty, just frightened, others mildly afflicted with dusty lung disease; fair numbers were grievously disabled, a few shortly died. These workers derived from scores of industries — foundries, potteries, mines, quarries, glass mills, natural stone grinding operations, sand blasting, soap factories — on and on.

Fifteen thousand workers in dusty trades have furnished fifteen thousand stories packed with drama, tragedy, fear, hysteria — and few with lying. A single one, shorn of all medical technicalities, is reassembled for sharing with those who elect an acquaintance with "silicosis."

MARTIN FORT is dead now and cannot speak for himself. I speak for him, using at times his own words:

"I am fifty years old now. For thirty-one years I have been a millstone sharpener. These stones are two kinds; both grind grain. They are granite, but we call them 'burr' (buhr) stones. That's what my dad called them. He worked here before me. He taught me this work. He was killed twenty years ago. A stone fell over on him. That was before we had cranes. I must have trimmed over twenty thousand stones, me and some other fellas; mostly the same wheels over and over. There are hundreds of them in the mill. When they get too thin, we throw them away. They are hauled out to the dump. In about four months' time they won't cut the grain right. Then they come in where I work. We rough 'em up first, then fine tool 'em. Years ago all the work was hand; now we have power tools."

"That's fine about the job, Martin," I encouraged, "but how about the dust?"

"Plenty of grit and chips all the time but not much dust. No clouds of dust 'cept when we blowed off the wheel." That fits into the picture, for the dust that causes silicosis is so fine that it cannot be seen with the naked eye.

Martin, a little short of breath, continued, "Always we wore goggles on account of the grit, but at that I have scars on my eyeballs from them flying chips. They wanted me to wear a muzzle to breathe through. I tried more than one kind, but, Doctor, I just couldn't suck enough air. Them things ain't made right."

The time had come to put our history-getting trolley on another wire. I sought to steer Martin. "When was the very first that you had any trouble and what happened then and what happened next?"

"When I'd been at this job about nineteen years, I was thirty-eight, I began to wheeze a little. Before that I'd walk home every night. It got my wind. Had to quit walking. Somebody told me I had asthma. Maybe I did. At the shop I wasn't as good a man as you might think. They put in cranes and that helped some. It's never let up. By now I'm bad as a horse with the heaves. Can't get no air down on my lungs."

"Are you working now?"

"I go down every day, but I mostly sit. There are two other fellas doing most of the tool work."

There were many more questions, but some of the history may be left untold. We made dust counts in Martin's work room. Every foot contained many millions of silica particles too small to be seen. An x-ray of Martin's chest brought out a snowstorm in his lungs — a snowstorm of white scars. Little unharmed lung tissue was left for breathing. No wonder he couldn't get air into his lungs; there was no room. Martin had silicosis.

No more work. Martin lived six years more — in the hospital. Those were not happy years. There was then no real treatment for silicosis. There is now — at least a promising treatment.

What happened to Martin during all those years of work? He never knew. His was the suffering but not the understanding. You shall be told the basic facts.

When silica dust in large amounts is breathed and reaches the millions of cunning little air sacs where oxygen of the air passes into the blood, it is an unwanted visitor. The body's policemen come to the rescue. These policemen are large cells within the blood that move by their own power, like amoebae. They engulf the intruder and a half-dozen like him, and off they start through the body's highways to some one of its several graveyards for unwanted arrivals. All goes well unless there be too many silica particles and too many dust cell carriers. Then a traffic jam takes place, with no traffic regulator. Millions of cells pile up on other millions. Discouraged, they die; and the silica, slowly dissolving, provokes a highly specific scar tissue which replaces useful breathing tissue. The disease so produced is silicosis. That is what happened to Martin.

THIS is no rare medical happening — no medical curiosity. Thousands of cases have blackened industry's medical record. On a long time basis, the majority of cases probably never were attributed to work. Alongside these all-too-many genuine dusty lung cases, may be found about an equal number of records of frightened workers who believe, along with their not always admirable lawyers, that their lungs have been grievously damaged by dusts. Some have never been exposed to harmful dusts; some suffer from direful lung diseases unrelated to dusts as the cause; some just imagine a lot of symptoms. Since in our education, yours and mine, as industrial hygienists we must face the spurious along with the real, travel with me five hundred miles from Martin Fort's former workplace to a courtroom.

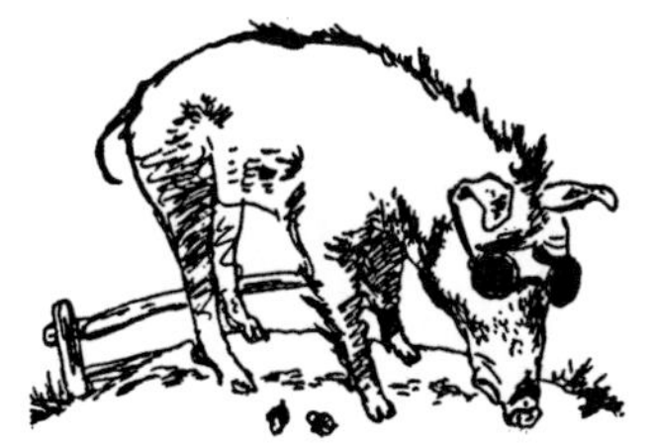

Chapter 7

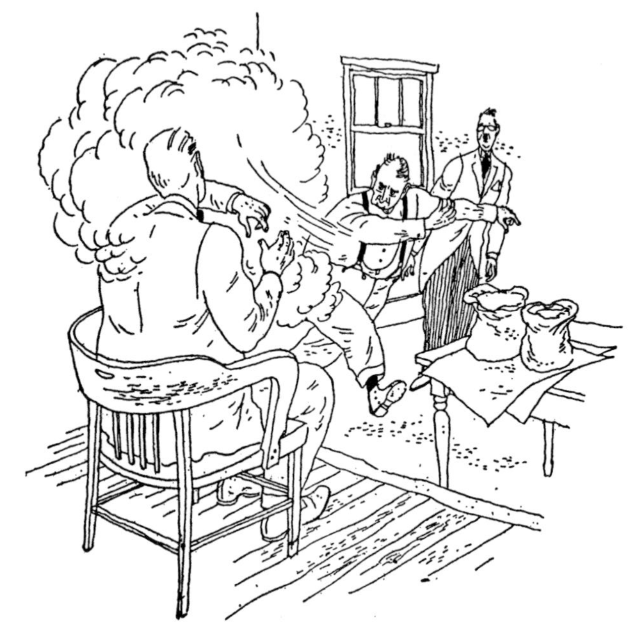

Trial by Dust

When the lights go out in factories, lights burn brighter in the courtrooms. Before the advent of unemployment insurance when depressions put brakes on the wheels of industry, men and women in desperation from empty pockets frequently turned on their employers, seeking to establish claims for all manner of trade diseases and injuries. Some of these claims were just and proper; the larger number rested heavily on imagination and cupidity.

In such times some lawyers and doctors likewise acquainted with cozenage, or possibly with empty waiting rooms, abetted workers in medical claims that to fairer men and women were preposterous.

Admirable lawyers have an ugly name for this unadmirable practice, "champerty"—the fomenting of litigation in order to share in any returns.

Forthright members of communities long have been concerned to see highly skilled physicians, hygienists, chemists, and engineers fervidly leagued with employers in the routing of legalistic onslaughts of claimants. "Why," they clamor among themselves, "is there no battery of equal talent standing by the side of the poor unfortunate victim?" To the initiated, the answer is so clear. Good claims seldom get into the courtroom. Promptly and fairly they are adjusted so soon as facts come to light. Scientists, having to live with themselves ever afterwards and to face their peers, scorn any share in champerty.

The softly sympathetic should not too greatly bemoan the plight of the plaintiff. In the hurly-burly football game of industrial injury litigation the plaintiff's kickoff is from any corporation's thirty-yard line. The less a witness knows, the more assertive and unqualified his testimony may be. Claimants frequently are surrounded by this sort of witness. Juries are strangely impressed by the sureness that emanates from unrecognized ignorance.

It has been my lot to spend many days in the witness chairs of many courtrooms; at times testifying for workers, at other times for trade unions, employers' trade associations, compensation boards, or medical societies—the doctor in the dock. That uneasy chair, dreaded by many as though it were the chair of electrocution, has been softened by many sittings until it is as comfortable as the chair before my breakfast table.

Spotted here and there in a long list of court cases dealing with dusts have been a number related to "tripoli." In a few areas of Missouri, Oklahoma, and Illinois are found scattered deposits of this uncommon mineral. This stone with its rich rose and yellow hues might well be used for building purposes in some places, but so great is its value that only a tycoon might dwell in a house so built. Instead, the mineral, properly ground and graded, finds its way into a score of industries — for buffing and polishing metal, for scouring, and as a filler in paints. In those states just mentioned there are a few factories wholly devoted to the preparation of this quarried product for industrial applications.

In one trial the plaintiff charged his employer with having operated the tripoli factory under conditions causing lung disease, disease in his case promising to prove fatal. While tripoli is a dusty material, it usually possesses peculiar electrostatic properties which operate to prevent any considerable dustiness of the atmosphere as breathed by workmen. Furthermore, the order of dustiness in any tripoli factory is low enough so that any industrialist with reasonable protective equipment in his plant may be assured of the absence of gross dust exposures. No less, the claim came.

One of the maneuvers of attorneys for plaintiffs was to seek a change of venue from more enlightened counties to backward localities where "flubdubbery" and "hokum" were usually more effective.

The particular trial which is here recorded was in a county so primitive as to be beyond the imagination of most urban dwellers. I shall refer to it as Fossil, a creation designed to evade the long arm of contempt of court from which this book might not be exempt. Since no railroad even skirted Fossil, it was reached by automobile on the morning of the trial. My breakfast was eaten off the counter of the local grocery store, with the grocer standing by, chatting amiably.

"Big day today," he offered.

"Really?" I managed.

"Yup. Big day. Biggest trial this here county ever had."

"Oh," I perceived, "a court case."

"Yup. Smartest lawyer in the county's going to make a monkey outen a big city corporation. Yup," he spat aimfully, "this here company's pretty nigh killed one of our boys — worked him in dust up to his neck. They're going to pay though. They're going to pay fifty thousand. This here lawyer's never lost a case yet."

"Really?"

"Nope — never lost a case. Say," he was inspired. "Say, you oughta stick around. My wife's coming down at nine o'clock for it. Fact is I'm going over myself. Wouldn't miss it."

"Well," I decided, "come to think of it, maybe I'll do just that."

In the courtroom there was no segregation of witnesses so that I, a prospective witness for the defense, was permitted to sit in on the trial. The homemade benches were hard and crowded. Only men graced the jury box, tanned, weather-beaten looking men, suggesting the hard-working farmer. Some were obviously unfamiliar with the razor as an article for everyday use. They were aware of their importance and ill concealed their admiration for the lawyer who was going to "twist the tail" of the big city corporation. He in turn was well aware of his jury, gloried in his awareness. When the jurymen had been sworn in, he removed his coat, the better to resemble their own overalled state. Later his tie came off, his shirt sleeves were rolled back, his chest was bared. He was a man of the people — or, specifically, of the jury. With a voice four times as loud as the courtroom demanded, he berated and derided the "wicked and vicious corporation that was making millions of dollars at the cost of lives of the country boys who became its slaves of employment." One member of the jury slyly winked his approval, while the audience scarcely suppressed its desire to cheer amid the pounding of the circuit judge's gavel.

The lawyer for the defense, however capable, was no master of the situation. He, as I, was as much out of place as an experimental physiologist at a ladies' anti-vivisection rally. Seeing the sartorial antics of his opponent, he felt called upon to do something. Whereupon he pulled up his shirt a little, pulled his tie askew and spat on the floor. It was not very effective.

As for the plaintiff, he was a sick man, desperately sick — of tuberculosis. His personal needs for money probably would not continue over any long period, and medically appraised it was dangerous to subject him to the ordeal of the trial. However, he coughed helpfully whenever his name was mentioned, and managed to give his testimony in whispers as he lay on his cot in the courtroom. No one could have doubted his own sincerity in believing that his employer had occasioned all of his ills. One look at him would have moved many juries to bring in a unanimously favorable verdict, regardless of testimony.

I was so wrapped up in the minute-by-minute happenings that hardly was there any time to appraise the utter ridiculousness of the procedure. Here was a jury of twelve men, little removed from illiteracy, who were to make a decision on a medical problem so intricate that at the time not more than twenty-five physicians in the entire country could have discussed it with authority. Here was a complex problem involving "phagocytosis," "lymphatic drainage," "x-ray shadows," "nodulation," "mottling," "the physics of electrostatic agglomeration," "the cryptocrystalline chemistry of tripoli." I felt none too sure of my own attainments, but the jury, good men and true, evinced no pain from any deficiencies.

The trial rolled on. It was a bit significant that the x-ray film purporting to be that of the patient made prior to his employment was not his at all, when compared with subsequent films produced after the arrival of far-advanced tuberculosis. Palpably this was true, but perhaps it represented more confusion than guile. Later, when it became apparent to the plaintiff's attorney that something was amiss, and that the something might be turned to good account for the defense, he sought permission from the court to withdraw the exhibit as having been included in error.

As the day wore on, the counsel for the accuser grew ever more adept in the art of becoming one with the jury. With touseled hair, wrinkled attire, and farmhand address he pleaded, exhorted, denounced, and accused in all the eloquence of a ham Shakespearean actor. One overheated juryman unselfconsciously removed his shoes during the proceedings. To the great delight of the country folk, the hero of the prosecution similarly disengaged his own footwear. Apparently it was to be a duel to the drawers.

The time came for me to take the stand as a witness late in the

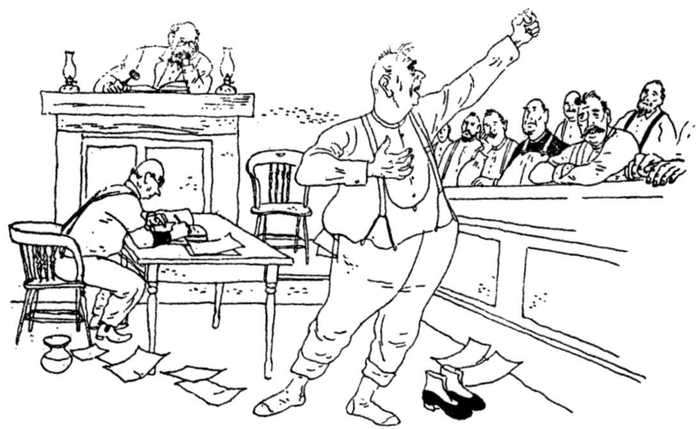

afternoon. An especial portion of the showman attorney's ire had been held in reserve for this moment and was about to burst the floodgates when a dramatic event occurred. I sometimes think, interrupting my direct testimony as it did, this incident may have determined the outcome of the trial. Two previous witnesses, one for either side, each of whom on the witness stand had been more than outspoken in his appraisal of the other, staged a fight in the courtroom. First there were only fists, but beneath whirling coats pistols suddenly glinted. The audience stampeded. The two opposing lawyers, all animosity temporarily forgotten, found refuge beneath the counsel table; the judge ducked beneath his bench, and I joined him there. Never before or since have I been on such intimate terms with a judge — a tangle of legs and arms in a common quest for safety.

Deputies stopped the fight with but a dash of blood spilled. The major trial was temporarily halted to hold a minor one. Since there was only one cell in the jail, one belligerent was locked up in the prosecuting attorney's office, lest there be a resumption of hostilities. The befuddled judge (provided this remark does not constitute contempt of court) conducted the secondary trial as an offense against the dignity of the court. After some testimony from each of the peace disturbers, or dignity destroyers, and the deputies who had separated them, the judge fined each disturber $8.25. Making sure his act was seen by the jury, each lawyer generously paid his partisan's fine, and the real business of the day was resumed.

After this interlude my testimony was anti-climax. The jury found itself without any interest in my descriptions of dusty lung diseases and how they differed from tuberculosis of the lungs. When the time came for his cross-examination of me, the lawyer for the plaintiff apparently sensed that too little of the spectacular was taking place. By the standards of that county I was too well dressed, and his agile brain was aware of an advantage to be gained.

"Look at this sleek man with his pretty clothes and his two dollar tie!" he screamed at the jury. "Look at his shoes! They must have cost fourteen dollars. He exemplifies the great wealth of this corporation," he ranted on. The jurymen shook their heads approvingly. "He makes more in one day for lying to save this corporation's dirty skin that you make in six months."

"We're going to make him look like us," yelled the attorney dramatically. I noted that by his side was a bag of tripoli dust. He reached into it for handfuls. "You say this dust is harmless," he growled at me, "Well then, take some for yourself," he exploded, showering me with the accumulation.

I took a lot of dust and wished for more. This indeed was poor strategy on his part. Meekly unprotesting, I gained a measure of sympathy. These people were thrifty folk, not quite seeing law or God's will in the useless soiling of a suit of clothes, nor seeing, even more importantly, any harm befalling me as I sat in a swirling cloud of the supposedly fatal dust. For my own part, I planned to send a cleaning bill to the allegedly wealthy corporation, the source of my discomfiture.

The lawyer's next move was to inquire whether I had the ability to read x-rays. Blinking dust from my eyes, I replied, "Yes, I have had some experience in radiology."

This was anathema. Whirling back to the jury he said triumphantly, "See, he's a radio announcer."

The jurymen stared blankly at me. I was dismissed with the plea that the jury take one last look at the "sleek, well-fed, hair-oiled, radio-announcing professional liar from Ohio."

At midnight the case went to the jury. The prosecuting attorney immediately ducked out to some clothing cache and returned no longer one of the people. Now he was the great lawyer awaiting the plaudits of his admirers, awaiting the inevitably favorable decision of the jury. His own hair was oiled. He had essayed the Champ Clark collar, donned his striped pants and long coat. Everyone shook his hand. On his face was a "Now-I-shall-run-for-Congress" expression.

The defense counsel was neglected. He had no back-slapping group of admirers about him. Utterly tired and a little haggard, as were all six of us representing the much berated corporation, he drifted over to me hoping for a word of comfort. I praised him for his intelligent handling of the case and his objectivity.

He said, "We really don't want to win this trial, even though the claim hasn't one iota of merit. We just don't want to lose. Winning would build up more ill will than the whole case is worth. The best thing would be a hung jury."

The weary audience stayed to a man. Among themselves they were betting ten to one that the plaintiff would win. The long delay, they explained, was due only to differences as to the amount of money to be awarded. For some technical legal reason, not within my ken, the clock was stopped just before twelve. Perhaps that maneuver saved one added day of jury pay. At two o'clock, by our own watches, an hour at which it was almost unbelievable that these eight-o'clock-retiring farmers could be at the courthouse, a worn jury returned to the courtroom. Discontent was obvious among them, and they seemed broken up into glowering factions. From all other portions of the courthouse the long-waiting spectators rushed back to the courtroom. The tired judge returned presently from his long wait in the sheriff's office. Instructing the jury as to procedure, he then inquired in utmost formality, "Gentlemen, have you reached a verdict?" Wearily the foreman got to his feet, "Your Honor," he replied, "we are unable to reach a verdict."

Uncomprehending silence — then with the same formality, the judge inquired, "Do you believe after further deliberation you might eventually reach a verdict?"

"There is no possible hope," the foreman answered glancing significantly at several of his fellow jurymen. The jury was dismissed. The trial was over.

I stood up, still brushing dust from my suit, and glanced fondly at the morose-looking jury. Maybe after all they hadn't been a bad lot. Yes, I'd quite underestimated them.

Chapter 8

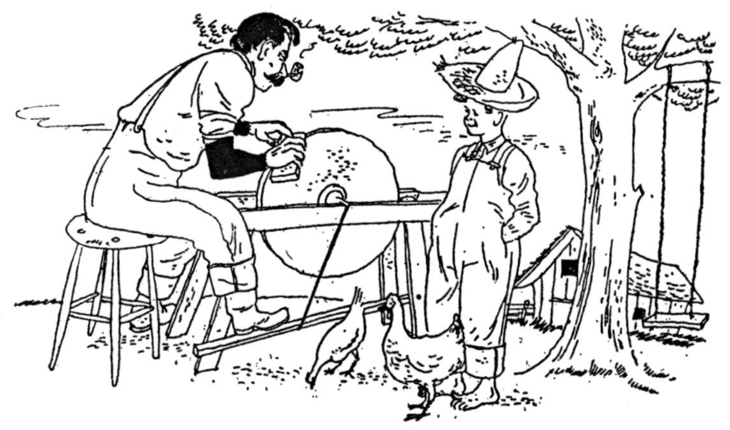

Two Ghosts of a City

AT THE END of any long court trial in which I have participated, win, lose, or draw, my customary reaction is an overwhelming desire to run away for two or three days and regain perspective lost in the tedious routine of courtroom procedure. At times trials involving occupational disease cases have lasted as long as thirty days, during which period the technical counselor is almost as much a prisoner as an arch criminal. He is constantly on demand, always in the courtroom awaiting the beckoning of attorneys bogged down in some medical intricacy, always available for conferences from breakfast to midnight, scarcely master of his own daily life. At the end, my S.D.W.P. (sense of duty well performed) regularly whispers, "Now you must take two or three days off." Such an instance prompted my first visit to Grindstone City, located at the thumb-nail tip of Michigan's mitten contour.

Casting a bass lure over a lake bottom covered with grindstones was a new experience. The bass refused to strike. My grizzled, be-whiskered old guide, Nelson, had a surplus of ready explanations.

"The wind's from the wrong direction, boss," he offered first. "Besides, there's no riffle on the water."

I grunted disgust.

"You should have been up here two weeks sooner," he mused wistfully. "Likely though, it'll be better this afternoon."

With this optimistic prophecy before me, fishing was temporarily foresaken. I asked a few questions about Grindstone City as we returned, perfunctory questions that drew voluble stories from the old man, who seemed to be the village historian. Eagerly he related the history of a century of grindstone manufacture.

Near 1835, into the town's small harbor sailed a sloop with Captain A. C. Peer in command. Captain Peer was looking for a cargo, and Grindstone City had just opened up a stone quarry. Captain Peer found no immediate cargo, but he founded an industry. He sensed that the rock of Grindstone possessed those unusual qualities required in the grinding of edged tools and cutlery. In 1838 Captain Peer built his first mill, a mill destined to furnish stones to Russia, China, Germany, and Japan, to furnish stones for industry everywhere, for farmers, for lumbermen, for housewives. A factor in the development of the entire Midwest, this Michigan pioneer industry had no provincial limitations. Its output reached the ports of the world.

Grindstone City is now but a monument to its former self. Its lake shores are lined with hundreds of culled stone discs, large and small, smooth and rough. Some of its few remaining walkways are paved with discarded grindstones and uncut slabs. Flower beds are edged with "kitchen stones" or waste stone cores. Outdoor tables are made of huge stone discs supported on stone legs. At the entrance to the now tiny village stands a large grindstone marker with the inscription, "In Memoriam of the Grindstone City Pioneers, 1835-1938."

WANDERING about the old quarries and mill sites are two ghosts. One is the ghost of the bygone industry itself, proud of its contributions to the world's growth and betterment, humble in its recognition of the superiority of those materials that supplanted it. The second ghost is furtive, little recognized, scarcely named, never praised—the ghost of a disease of stone workers produced by mill work.

Sandstone is abundant throughout the world, but few deposits possess the peculiar texture necessary for the grinding of edged tools and cutlery.

Coarse buhr and ganister stones may be used in the grinding of paint, corn, or wheat; but for a natural stone to be satisfactory for cutting edge production, the stone must present fine, hard granules of silica, strongly bonded with silicates, carbonates, and other minerals, particularly free from "hardheads" — embedded pebbles, immediately destructive of sharp edges.

Such a stone was discovered at least by 1835 on the shores of Lake Huron, but its distribution was limited to a few hundred acres. Enough stone was found at the site of Grindstone City to provide continuous operations over nearly one hundred years without exhausting the supply. Cooperating with Captain Peer were Messrs. Pease and Smith, who operated the first quarry. In later years, many other names appeared, including J. B. Johnson (1860), William H. Cooper (1865), Worthington and Sons (1871), the Lake Huron Stone Company, operated by the Wallace family, then in 1888 the Cleveland Stone Company. Regardless of owners or operators, the stone remained the same. Through "trenching," "drilling," "reaming," "blasting," "wedging," stone blocks were procured and hauled to the mills. There the big rocks were "eyed," "chipped," "scabbled," and "dressed" into industrial grindstones for farmers and lumbermen — in endless profusion. In early days all work was done by hand. In time came gang saws, powered chisels, rim cutters. The earlier square, hand-cut eyes were replaced by circular eyes, cut by coring machines. Though the trade was essentially seasonal, limited to warmer months, some work was carried on throughout the year.

In a good year as much as twenty-five thousand tons of stones were shipped by sailboat, steamer or rail. Some of these stones were seventy-two inches in diameter and fourteen inches in thickness. Stones of the best grade commanded a price of $15.00 to $18.00 per ton, and single stones at times weighed as much as three tons.

In the mills and in the quarries, one hundred and fifty workers were employed; but in the course of nearly one hundred years of activity, the aggregate of workers represented a few thousand. Here in these quarries and mills workers gained their livelihood; some aged and died, some died prematurely, but all contributed to the development and progress particularly of this country's Midwest section but also, in some measure, to the industries of the world.

Much of this we later learned from old Angus McCachen, the works foreman, just a few months before his death. Tottering on feeble legs, he led us to the former site of the mill, the power house, the storage yard, the docks, the railroad station. This aged Scotsman, refusing to recognize his industry as dead, continued to live in a tiny house at the edge of his former domain.

"You just wait. You'll see the return of the grindstone industry. I won't be here. I'll be dead."

For many years Grindstone City thrived. "Then," to quote one of the surviving operators, Mr. Lee Wallace, "about 1900 there came a rumor that an artificial abrasive had been discovered. At that time we didn't think it would amount to much. But it did."

This statement sent me away to libraries, hunting up the history of that synthetic material that proved the ruin of the grindstone industry.

In the midst of years of prosperity, the anlage of the destroyer of the natural abrasive stone as a major agent in industry already existed. Just as the germ of the ultimate destructive agent of the human body long and quietly may reside within an organ or tissue, awaiting the pathologic "Der Tag," so the substance destined to

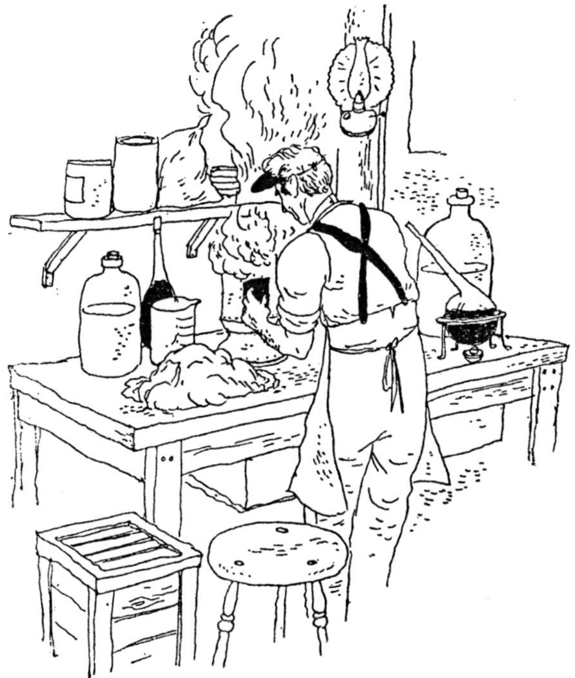

reduce the natural grindstone industry to comparative obsolescence existed long before the years of its triumph.

The year was 1891, the place Monongahela, Pennsylvania. There, in a makeshift laboratory, a then unknown chemist endeavored to make artificial diamonds from clay and coke in an electric furnace, improvised from a plumber's solder pot. No diamonds appeared in the pot, but something perhaps even more valuable — a few highly-colored, iridescent crystals. A successful failure, these synthesized crystals proved to be harder than any known substance and usable in cutting any precious stones, including diamonds. Believing the substance to represent a mixture of carbon and corundum, its discoverer, Edward G. Acheson, created the term "carborundum." So small was the early yield that carborundum was protected as though itself a precious stone. On a petty scale it was peddled to lapidaries and jewelers, with the carat as the unit of sale and at a price equivalent to $880.00 per pound. Then came patents, corporations, fame, and fortunes. Recent years have seen the yearly production of thirty thousand tons of carborundum, obtainable at fifteen cents per pound.

Out of that pot came today's metal fabrication industry as best exemplified by automobile manufacture. In this one industry more than two hundred operations include high-speed grinding as an essential step. Romance in a plumber's pot! It may be improper to label this pot as the mother of mass production, but it would be foolish to deny it a place near to parenthood.

Not solely to carborundum may be attributed the industrial revolution built around synthetic abrasives. Emery is a non-identical twin. Carborundum never has been found as a natural mineral; emery is widely distributed over the earth. Pliny, the Roman, knew of the abrasive action of emery, which he designated "naxium." When the Bible refers to "adamant," emery possibly is the substance described. In 1830, a railroad was under construction from Boston to the Hudson River. In a cut near Chester, Massachusetts, emery was found in some abundance. Natural emery is aluminum and iron oxides together with impurities. The Chester discovery first was believed to represent iron, as emery was then little known. Blast furnaces were created to smelt iron. Dismal failure was the lot of the promoters, since emery does not lend itself to any such enterprise. Years later these deposits were worked as a source of a natural abrasive but soon lost their importance, for in 1899 Charles B. Jacobs produced synthetic emery from bauxite.

The mere existence of carborundum and emery is not sufficient for industries' requirements; grinding wheels were the need. Abrasives in granular form may be bonded in a score of fashions, each meeting some especial demand. Carborundum and emery, in their many modifications, shapes, sizes, granular sizes, fulfill the great majority of industry's needs for high speed mineral abrading.

Boon that these twins were and are to industry, they proved iniquitous to Grindstone City and to all grindstone cities.

It is fairly easy to fix the moment of death of an observed person, difficult to fix the death of an industry. When did the whaling industry of New England die, if in fact it is dead? When died the buggy industry? When died natural grindstone manufacture? Quite bravely, but a little wistfully, grindstone producers point to a few evidences of virility, the dependence of some few industries on natural stones, the continued operation of several abrasive stone quarries. Just as carborundum and artificial emery ended the widespread use of natural stones for grinding, so the coming of concrete largely terminated the profitable operation of sandstone quarries for building-stone purposes. Carborundum, emery, and Portland cement have turned rock quarries into fish ponds. The small farm is the residual stronghold of the natural grindstone, but unlike a bar of soap a single grindstone may last for generations. A pat simile is, "As lasting as a farmer's grindstone."

Acheson, poking around in his plumber's crucible in 1891, mortally wounded Grindstone City. On September 29, 1929, Grindstone City gave up the struggle. Gone are the quarries' activities, tripods and drills — gone are the powder cans — gone are the trams — gone are the gang saws — gone are the cranes — gone are the docks — gone are the sailing vessels and steamers — gone is the railroad — gone are Grindstone's workers.

When an inquiry was made as to the whereabouts of the quarry and mill workers, a few remaining elders of the village replied, "Most of the mill hands died of 'grit consumption.'" Some used other terms, "dust on the lungs," "rock tuberculosis," "grinders' consumption." Others said, "A lot of the mill hands died of some curious disease that the doctors said came from the dust."

HERE, then, is Grindstone City's second product — silicosis. Long before the term "silicosis" was utilized in 1870 by Visconti, these quarries were turning out silica grindstones by the thousands. The all-embracive term for dusty lung diseases, "pneumoconioses," was not devised by Zenker until that same year. The x-ray, indispensable in the diagnosis of silicosis during life, was not discovered until 1895 by Roentgen in Germany. Not until many years thereafter did the services of the roentgenologists extend to such places as Grindstone City.

There is then no cause for wonder that nowhere are there available precise medical records of dusty lung diseases among Grindstone City's workers. No ancient vital statistics for the State of Michigan revealed any high incidence of silicosis or tuberculosis in the Grindstone City area. Gone are the physicians who treated these ailing workers.

Not even the most critical may condemn these pioneer manufacturers for any negligence in the safeguarding of their workers. If there was no medical lore for the guidance of physicians, how much less may it be believed that any awareness might have been the lot of the manufacturers. To their credit it may be pointed out that in the quarries all drilling was by wet methods, thus preventing much dust formation, although wet drilling doubtless represented a desirable trade practice rather than any foresight in worker protection. No less, it is not known that any silicosis arose among quarriers. Further to the credit of these manufacturers is it that attempts were made to remove dust produced in the mills. Unconscious protection was provided through the performance of stone dressing in open sheds, while the limiting of most mill operations to six months of the year was another unplanned but no less life-saving feature of the work.

Just as Grindstone City's major product, grindstone, travelled to many places over the world, so the second product, silicosis, appeared in far-flung places. Among many other applications, natural grindstones are used in the edging of axes. In Bolles' "Industrial History of the United States" (1878) there appears an engaging description of the axe industry in America. Some of its tragic description is here repeated:

"The next stage in the progress of the axe toward completion brings us to the grinding and polishing departments. Some idea of the relative importance of this branch of the manufacture may be had from the fact that it costs $100 worth of grindstones daily to bring the axes to the marketable stage, to say nothing of the immense expenditure of energy in polishing afterwards. Huge stones from Nova Scotia and the West lie about the shipyards full 7 feet in diameter, many of them; and in no longer than three weeks' time they are used up. Many of the men ride on 'horses' while grinding, thus enabling them to bring their whole bodily avoirdupois to aid the process of abrasion, while the fine dust flies in clouds from the stones in every direction, notwithstanding the stones are all the time completely deluged with water.

"The men in this section are from their peculiarly hazardous work, ruled out of all the life insurance companies; since the constant inhalation of the grit and bits of steel thrown off in the process induces the 'grinders' consumption,' as it is rightly termed, from which a premature death is rarely averted. It is said that Americans will not work in these rooms, which are filled by French Canadians, who stop a few years, and then go home to linger a while and die."

Reference to huge stones from the "West" may refer to Grindstone City stones, but this is not known. Years later (1920) another observer of grinders' consumption in the axe grinding industry, noted as a "hotbed" of silicosis, included in his report this letter:

"I have seen quite a number of cases of so-called grinders' consumption. The symptoms are excessive shortness of breath on slight exertion, dry cough, and great prostration. The grinders are from the Polanders and Finns for the past dozen years. The disease takes hold of them more frequently and is more rapidly fatal than among the grinders of former years and of other nationalities. When I came here forty years ago I found the victims among the Yankees who had ground some twenty years before. These could grind eighteen or twenty years before having to give up. The French-Canadians were then grinding. They could work twelve to sixteen years. They became frightened off and the Swedes took up the work. They would get the disease in eight or ten years. Now the Finns and Polanders are at it, and they last only three to five years, and the disease is more common among them."

Some idea of the quantity of dust formerly produced in grinding with natural silica grindstone may be gained from this statement:

"A stone of 72 inches in diameter weighs approximately two tons. One 84 inches across weighs three tons. Stones vary greatly in thickness, viz., from 8 to 13 inches, an axe or a tool stone usually being about 11 inches, while that used for machetes is about 13 inches wide. A stone 70 inches by 12 inches, used to grind axes and tools, will last about one month, while that used for machetes will last three months. Stones are discarded when they reach a diameter of 29 inches. From forty to fifty stones on an average are used up each month throughout the year."

WITHOUT condemnation, solely as an act of the historian, it is recorded that the manufacturers of natural silica grindstone everywhere, without guile or evil design, may have furnished many workers over the world a work material that insidiously brought about the end of their days. Thus some of both the makers and users of these stone wheels apparently were destroyed by this king of occupational diseases — silicosis.

Happier are work conditions attending many of today's dusty trades. Dust-producing machines and operations are likely to be surrounded by exhaust systems that maintain dust concentrations below dangerous thresholds. The quantity of dust present in the air may be measured by cunning instruments that permit the counting of each particle. Various substances may be added to silica to render it less injurious. Essentially all grinding is carried out with carborundum or other synthetic abrasives, the dusts of which are almost entirely inert. X-ray examinations of the chests of workers may reveal the early beginnings of dusty lung diseases. Comparatively few workers in all the United States are now wholly unprotected against the ravages of silica dust. The grindstone makers in Michigan and elsewhere, working before the days of x-rays, dust counts, petrographic microscopes, adequate respirators and efficient dust arresters — in fact, before the day of any scientific knowledge of silicosis — furnished a part of the doleful experience that makes occupational disease exposures no longer tolerable.*

If you would learn the history of an old and small manufacturing plant, your best bet is to stay away from the front office and the minutes of directors' meetings. Instead, hunt up the "Old Timer,"

* Republished from *Hygeia* with the approval of the American Medical Association.

the worker "legacy." Nearly every old plant has at least one. Their temporal bench mark is commonly the Chicago World's Fair or the Spanish-American War. One such patriarch, afflicted with "galloping" garrulity, from whom I sought the dust disease history of a pottery, poured out instead that which now is recorded. This possibly belongs only in the apocrypha.

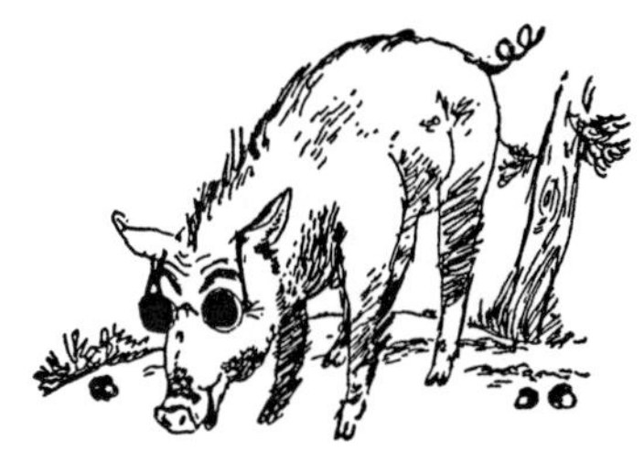

Chapter 9

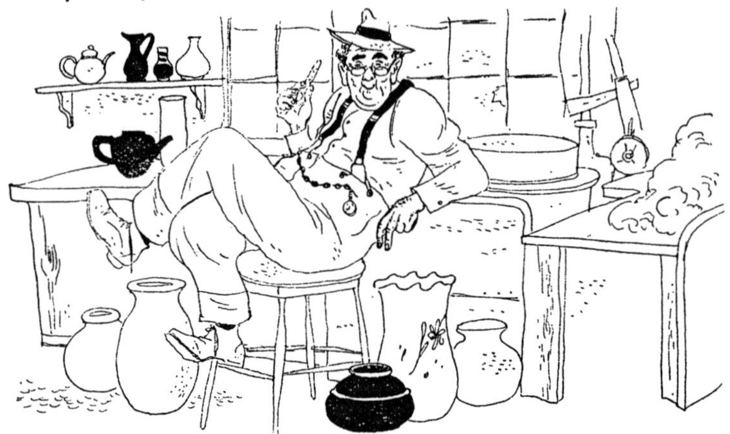

Amateur Versus Expert Pottery Making

At one time I held sixty-seven jobs simultaneously. That may sound Thrasonic, but the facts belie any occasion for gasconading. These, apart from two or three substantial ones, were casual, representing employing groups that leaned on me for services only when the threatening hand of occupational diseases clutched some workers. There were almost as many titles as there were jobs. This immaterial multiplicity included "Consultant," "Adviser," "Referee," "Visiting Physician," "Industrial Hygienist," "Lecturer," "Professor"— and sometimes just "The Doc."

One of these long past connections was with a pottery. Here it was that I met Newt, the night watchman. It is possible that if Newt had a birth certificate it would have shown "Newton" as the given name, but few times thereafter was he other than "Newt," although, if his name was for the moment forgotten, he became "that two-fingered night watchman."

Newt became more than my admirer, almost my slave, when I cured his deafness. For several years he had been shut off from all but the loudest sounds about him; fearing all medical service, he had patiently accepted his affliction without any aural examination. As part of a routine physical examination, I discovered that his ear canals merely were packed full and hard with ear wax. After some days of softening with mild alkalies and with glycerin, it was possible to flush out of these canals chunks of grumous ear wax. Then Newt heard as well as any person of his age.

Being night watchman gave Newt scant claim to any artisanship as a potter, but when he learned that I had set up a potter's wheel in my barn he was among the first to volunteer as a counsellor, helper, and occasional source of materials. Thereby he fell into a guileless snare of my making. The aged Newt was the plant's "remembrancer." Newt's theme phrase was "I recollect when." I wanted to know about medical affairs in early days; Newt's registry of the pottery's past seemed to have a gap for anything medical, but I learned everything else.

As the months went by and the number of pieces on the shelf above the horse trough increased, Newt, with justification, became critical of their quality.

"This," he said, "doesn't come up to them fine pieces in the display rooms."

I could but agree, but I pointed out that that pottery had been in existence for many tens of years and that some of the best artists in the country had decorated those pieces. To this Newt objected, pointing out,"The very best pieces up there were not made by the artists at all. Just go up and try to buy one of these pieces of 'Firefly' pottery that sits up in the museum section. The lady up there will be very polite, and she will tell you that those pieces are not for sale — that they are museum specimens. Then if you go ahead and ask her if she could make up a special piece, she'll tell you that the pottery for many years had not made that 'Firefly' pottery, but that ain't the whole truth. They can't make that pottery no more. They don't know how. It just happened by accident, and they don't know what the accident was. I was there when the accident happened. Would you like to hear about that?"

"I would."

"Don't ever tell anybody that I told you this story, and if you ask any of the bosses around the plant if what I say is true, they will tell you that it is all a damned lie, but it ain't. It's Bible truth."

At this point Newt interrupted to inquire about the best treatment for a boil on the cheek, saying that his "old lady" had one. Before I could make any reply, he launched into his own therapeutics, giving as his opinion that a poultice of soft sheep manure drew the "beelin" to a head quicker than anything else. When I pointed out with utter scorn the folly of any such treatment, his medical dignity was hurt and he threatened to go home before I got the "Firefly" pottery story. One of my best cigars mollified him, and he started his account of the famous "Firefly" pottery, known to many museums where ceramics are collected.

"It was in the dead of winter more than twenty years ago. All day long pottery had been set with care in the saggers and later in the kiln. I wasn't there, I was the night watchman, but I knowed that's what happened. They always did it that way. Toward night the fires were started up. In those days we always fired with coal. Jake Folsom was the night kiln fireman. He was late that night, which is lucky, because he was already drunk. If he had come on before the superintendent left, he never would have been allowed to stay. Already a big fire was going, but Jake shoveled on more coal. Soon he went across the street to the bar, and when he came back the fire didn't need no more coal, but he put on more. I said, 'Jake, you're going to catch hell for ruining all that pottery.'

"Jake said, 'I might as well catch hell as to freeze to death.' So he put on more coal. Then he went back to the saloon. It was none of my business to pay any attention to the kiln fire except to see that none of the buildings were set on fire. After a while Jake came back and put on some more coal. This was the biggest, hottest fire I ever

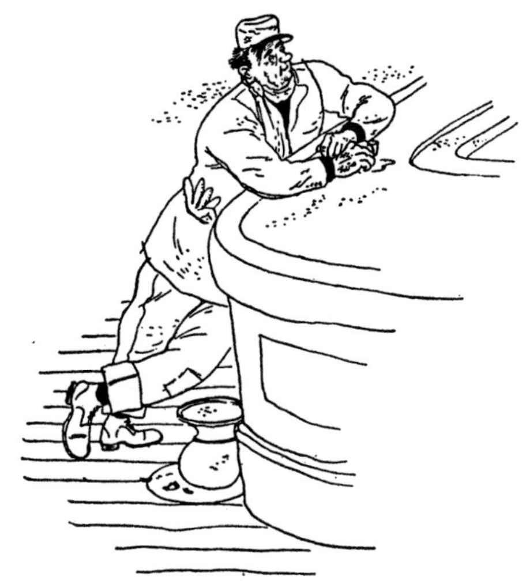

saw in any kiln. The bricks on the outside were red hot, and you could see all sorts of melted drippings off the saggers. Jake was crazy drunk then and threatened to hit me with a shovel when I told him that what he was doing wasn't right. The next time Jake went to the saloon, he never came back at all. That night the weather was so cold that the saloon never did close up. They knew that if they put out all those drunken bums some of them would freeze to death before they got home.

"That there kiln pretty near melted down. The next morning there was hell on all sides. I stayed around to see what was going to happen. The superintendent came in, and he was wild. He knew that all that pottery must be ruined. He was the boss, and he'd get blamed. He asked me what Jake had done, but I said I didn't know, as I was just making my rounds as night watchman, punching the clock. About that time somebody said that Jake was still over in the bar. The boss went over and right there fired Jake. Two or three of the boys sort of helped him over to the pay office, and they cashiered him that minute. When the big office bosses came, the superintendent went up and got them. They were mad too. Everybody came down to have a look — even the artists. They were put out because they said some of the best pieces that had ever been made was in that lot.

"The superintendent got some of the boys and began to clear out the kiln. Most of the saggers and everything in them were just flattened out like molasses candy before you start to pull it. Everything looked ruined. A lot of it was so melted together that before they could get it out they had to jimmy it with crowbars. It was worse on the outside than the inside. Long before noon they were getting close to the middle when the superintendent says, 'What's this?'

"And there was the prettiest piece of pottery that anybody ever saw. Nobody had ever made any pottery like that. It looked as though you could see through it, but you couldn't see through it. It looked as though you were seeing deep down in the pottery and way down in there were hundreds of lightnin' bugs, all of them lit up. The superintendent told the boys to wait. He got the big bosses again. They saw this one piece of pottery and their eyes nearly popped out. They looked in to see if there were any more good like that, and sure enough they could see that right in the middle of the kiln there was going to be a lot of this fancy pottery. Everybody got excited again. Careful-like they took out every piece, so as not to break any.

"The sales manager says, 'We'll sell all the pottery like this you can make.'

" 'We'll make some more all right,' says the superintendent.

"I left then; so what happened after that I only know from what other folks told me. They got about one hundred pieces of this fancy pottery. As good luck would have it, the biggest pieces had been put in the middle of the kiln; so nearly all of these fine pieces were big pieces. That was lucky the way things turned out.

"Then they sent for Jake. Jake was still drunk and couldn't tell them much. He never did recollect what happened. That night they was waiting for me. First I told them I hadn't seen a thing. Then when they told me they wanted to make more of this pottery and wanted to find out just what had happened, I told them everything. They didn't blame me none. I didn't have a single drink that night anyway. Right away next day they hired Jake again, and they told him to do just what he did; but Jake never had any remembrance of what he had done. Then they told me to stick by Jake and tell him what to do and about how much coal to put on, but they never could make any more pottery like that.

"All the officials had a meeting, and they called this pottery 'Firefly' pottery. Then they began to hold exhibits all over the country and in other countries too. They took all the prizes. They sold some of the pieces — mostly to museums — and got big money for them. When anybody else wanted to buy a piece, they always was told these pieces mostly were made for museums. The real reason is they don't know how to make that pottery. They tried everything. They never told anybody about all this being just an accident, but all the old timers around here know. Maybe I shouldn't be telling you, Doc, about this, you bein' a newcomer. Don't ever tell anybody I told you, but someday you just go up to that lady and tell her you want to buy a piece of 'Firefly' pottery and see what she tells you."

"Fine, Newt. With all that happened, maybe you got a second or third — some piece that was just 'Firefly' on one side and something else on the other."

"No, I didn't, Doc, but down at my house I have the piece of pottery that took the first prize in Paris at that big Fair. That goes way back years, and that pottery isn't much compared to this 'Firefly' pottery. Besides, they only gave it to me because it is cracked on one side. They never keep any piece of pottery that ever won a prize if it even gets nicked a litttle bit, so they gave it to me; and, Doc, since you fixed up my ears, that gives me an idea. I'd like to give that piece of pottery to you to put along here with your trash. If you keep the good side front, it will look all right. Besides, even if it was cracked on both sides it would look better than your pottery."

Newt kept his word. To this day I have the piece of pottery that Newt claimed took first prize in Paris. That's the way of investigative work. Here I started out to learn about "potter's rot" — silicosis of the pottery variety and ended up with little more than a cracked bit of pottery. But many another questing has ended even more barren.

My own puerile pottery making never reached any high estate. Once my ego was dilated when point-blank I was refused admission to a pottery in Zanesville, Ohio, on the plea that I was competitor. The little time available for pottery puttering was spent in seeing other and better potters at work. This travel took me to Central America to see the crude pottery of the Maya. Soon, I found myself more engrossed in the occupational diseases of those strange lands. In Quintana-Roo, I found an ancient disease, frequently depicted on Mayan pottery hundreds of years old, in a new guise — an old disease now to be added to the category of occupational diseases.

Chapter 10

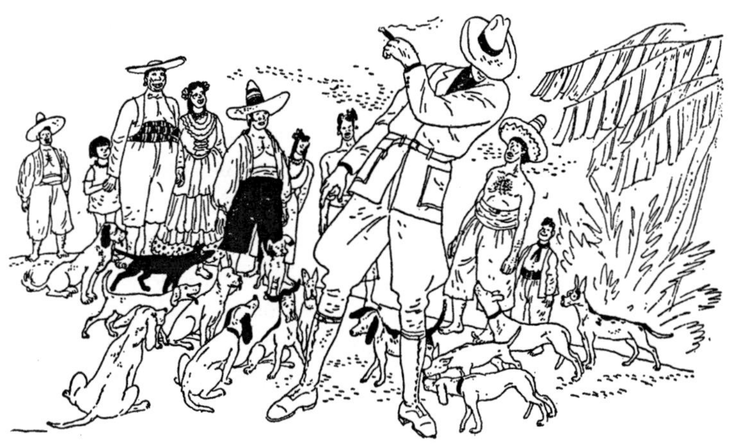

Jungle Ulcer

HOWEVER primitive an industry may be, occupational diseases seem inevitable. I have seen such diseases among copra collectors in tropical countries, copra being the dried meat of the cocoanut, and among sisal makers on Middle American haciendas. In Guatemala I have found lead poisoning among Indians using lead for glazing native pottery. Once in Yucatan I was afforded opportunity to investigate one occupational disease that afflicts the collectors of chicle. Here is the story:

This started in Merida at the Grand Hotel. Merida is no jungle city — instead a cultured and wealthy city of magnificent homes, thousands of windmills, underground rivers, music, soft-spoken Spaniards, endless drinks, a city surrounded by haciendas, a vast acreage of henequen. Merida is the chicle capital of Yucatan as well as the political capital of the State. Here it was I found Manuel, the news agency's representative.

Manuel made a little oration. "You, Doctor, are an investigator of occupational diseases. You have told us stories of occasional cases of arsenic poisoning in your great factories in the United States, of benzol poisoning, of deafness from noise. You really have never seen occupational diseases by the thousand. If you would see endless cases of an occupational disease, you should go to the jungle and see the chicleros."

"Well, what do these chicleros show as a disease?"

"Their ears drop off, holes appear in their cheeks, their eyelids are eroded, deep sores appear on their chins, their necks and their arms. If you really would be of service to workers, if you really want to do something for Yucatan, find out what it is that afflicts the chiclero. Nobody knows."

That was a challenge.

Manuel was wrong when he said no one knew about the disease of chicleros. Admirable descriptions even then had been provided by Shattuck and his associates in his book, "The Peninsula of Yucatan," and afterwards in his book "A Medical Survey of the Republic of Guatemala." Morley, the archaeologist extraordinary of Yucatan, is well familiar with this disease, in both its modern and prehistoric aspects. On occasion, at his hacienda at Chichen Itza, he described to me the excavation of figurines of prehistoric Maya showing deformed ears, not unlike the ears of the afflicted chicleros.

Neither of these investigators was concerned with this disease as one related to occupation. Able as were their thoughts, they were not translated into terms of "the little piece of man" in a commercial product. To them, this was only an ancient and modern tropical disease.

Not for three years was there opportunity to accept Manuel's challenge. For the anthropologist, the archaeologist, the ethnologist, the mahogany logger, the chiclero, penetration of the jungle is all in the year's work. For a physician who had never seen a jungle, whose entire medical activities were surrounded by hospitals, specialists, consultants, laboratory facilities at his beck and call, the prospect of going, and going alone, into the jungle was terrifying. It was done, but not as a magnificent Stanleyesque safari with porters, pack trains, tents, guns or tom-toms. It was the puny sort of expedition that outrages the archaeologist, puts tongues in cheeks, and lifts eyebrows.

First to the port of Progreso in Yucatan, out of New Orleans, on the little Norwegian henequen freighter "Bertha Brovig," with the genial Captain Hanson and his comforting supply of habanero. Thence to Merida for a saturation with quinine and typhoid vaccine, the accumulation of a few essential supplies, hammocks and bedding, anti-venins for the possible snake-bite, microscopes, stains, slides, canteens, water jugs, canned foods, camera supplies — notebooks.

To the would-be investigator bent on getting into the jungle to the very source of the disease, it was both gratifying and deflating to find that the most severe cases of the chiclero's occupational disease are now brought for treatment by plane from the jungle outposts to the modern hospitals at Merida.

Helpful and cooperative were Drs. Villamil and Arjona, outstanding physicians of Merida. These physicians assembled cases of chiclero's disease in their offices for demonstration. Their files afforded many case histories and photographs. Through their microscopes, the causative organisms of the disease were seen in abundance. Under their praiseworthy treatment, it was possible to see active lesions checked within a few days; but no treatment will replace a destroyed ear, or hide the scars of multiple ulcers.

Still there were mysteries. These physicians offered no explanation why only chicleros are commonly involved, why the chiclero does not communicate his disease to members of his family after his sojourn in the jungle, why residents at the jungle's edge almost never acquire the disease unless at some time they enter the jungle. They offered no information as to the mechanism of the transmission of the disease from one person to another. They recounted endless variations of legendary stories about a biting fly that lives under the wings of the wild turkey, or the native bustard, or the water heron. They related equally engaging stories about the acquisition of the disease from the peccary or the jungle deer, or from plants.

With scientific straightforwardness, they displayed their crossed fingers with all of these narrations and shook their heads in eloquent disbelief of their reliability.

Through good fortune, a group of semi-official motion picture photographers from Mexico City were present in Merida to photograph the sports activities featured in the dedication of a great stadium for that portion of communistic Mexico. While many unkind things have been said about the machinations of that regime in Mexico, nothing but praise may be extended to their motion picture photography of chiclero's disease. These films, made on patients brought to Merida, and carried to the States for development, were pronounced by the Eastman Kodak Company to be superb examples of medical photography. The anticipated hardships of the jungle life were fast scattering.

To the would-be explorer, it was further discomfiting to gain the report that in the dry season numerous cases of chiclero's disease might be found in almost any village, among the chicle gatherers lately returned from the tall brush. Since our investigation was made just at the transition from the wet to the dry season, it was pointed out to us that it would be possible both to visit villages, questing for cases, and also to go to the jungle where some camps were still in operation. Both were done.

While residents of Merida live almost at the rim of the jungle, to them it is scarcely more real than hell, Atlantis, or the Patagonian Islands. Only from archaeologists, chicle executives and plane operators was it possible to obtain any substantial information about the land, people, and threats of the jungle. In preparation for my trip, I pieced together much information, familiarity with which might be helpful in following later happenings.

Jungles, Indians, prehistoric ruins, swamps, hordes of insects —

of such is the land of chicle and the chiclero. These lands are found in Yucatan, Quintana-Roo, the Peten part of Guatemala, British Honduras. Other portions of the semitropics in truth do furnish some chicle. The chicle gatherers — the chicleros — live in scores of villages, fewer towns and rare cities in higher lands apart from the inhospitable jungles. Before the rainy season comes and the sap flows in the sapote trees, the chiclero bundles up a change of clothing, straps on his machete, leaves behind his wife and children, and penetrates the jungle for a seven-month work period of unbelievable hardship, exposure and productivity. Even to those chicleros who have spent forty years in the jungle, every additional season promises newness and uncertainty.

No ordinary man is this chiclero. He boasts, "You have to be half-man and half-peccary to get along in the jungle."

Some of the chicle-bearing countries teem with the stocky, sturdy, muscular Maya Indians; but as a rule they are not sufficiently hardy to become chicleros. Any assemblage of chicleros defies anthropological classification. They represent undelineable mixtures of Maya, Yaqui, Aztec, Carib, Negro, and Caucasian. In Yucatan and Quintana-Roo the greater number are referred to as mestizos, which properly describes the mixture of Maya and Spanish blood. By consent, anyone who is neither Spanish nor Maya among chicleros, is a mestizo.

Whatever may be their racial origin, these chicleros share many qualities — apparent immunity to many diseases, the ability to drink with impunity water that would lay low the average person in three days' time, a willingness to accept a diet deficient in every respect, acceptance of work in daily pouring rains, capacity to survive in a jungle without roof overhead, bed under body, or shoes under foot. These chicleros join in another common quality — an utter disbelief that over the world there could possibly be enough people to chew the twelve million pounds of chicle they yearly produce. They believe that secretly the greater portion must be turned into some mysterious munitions, or made into automobiles or clothing. The temptation is to forget about chicleros as patients and write about chicleros as chicleros.

Chicle, the base of chewing gum, is the sap or resin of the tree that the native Mayan calls the yaa. To the better informed it is the sapote, zapote or sapodilla. This evergreen tree grows by the millions in the jungles of the areas mentioned. The natives believe that the supply is inexhaustible, but this belief is not shared by visiting foresters who predict the inevitability of exhaustion through wastage. The chiclero attaches at the base of every tree to be tapped a small fabric or rubber sac. Then with his machete he slashes the coarse bark in a series of irregular V's, from ten to twenty-four inches apart, on one side of the tree, as he climbs upward. Tapping begins at daylight and continues only until mid-morning. The sap flows immediately, and the flow is completed by nightfall. Not for five to eight years may this tree again be slashed. Thousands die. The viscous sap that flows into the bag is the starting point of chewing gum. It is transported to the centrally located boiling kettles, reduced to proper consistency, shaped in wooden molds into bricks or marquetas. The chicle is now ready for shipment.

Chicle camps range in population from one hundred to nine hundred workers. The common number is about three hundred. The sites of these camps may be changed from year to year as the supply of trees becomes locally exhausted. As the work radiates from the central camps, numerous smaller camps spring up scattered over many square miles. No buildings are erected beyond a few thatched roofs supported on poles over the meager supplies and the euphemistic "office" of the "boss chiclero." Most of the workers are tree slashers, a few tend the concentration kettles, a few are muleteers for the pack trains, and a very few are the hunters who seek to supply the camp with peccary meat, wild turkey, deer, and the edible flesh of other jungle animals.

Through a generous arrangement of nature, the very tree that is tapped for chicle also furnishes the chiclero's chief jungle fruit. This succulent sapodilla plum, found in three colors of pulp, white, pink, and smoky grey, is, apart from sunshine, the chiclero's bulwark against avitaminoses.

When one sees the hardiness of the chiclero, living chiefly on a diet of black bean soup and tortillas, he begins to wonder about the barrage of insistence upon artificial vitamin consumption in other parts of the world. While the mouth-agape visitor returns to the States and boasts over the terrible hardships of sleeping in a hammock, the chiclero yearns for that day when he may be so affluent as to possess a hammock. He sleeps on the ground, if he may find a dry spot. At the beginning of the rainy season few insects are present. As the rains progress, swarming insects in endless variety seem to double their population daily — insects that bite, sting, feed, crawl — insects by day, even more by night — noisy insects, colored insects, large and small, mites, midges, flies and bees. Except for the boss chiclero, mosquito nets are almost as foreign as to Antarctica. The chiclero in the jungle "takes" whatever comes. There are no luxuries in a chicle camp.

In an earlier day, the chicle workers, after their work's seasonal holiday of five months, assembled in many groups several days before the coming of the rainy season in villages near to the jungle's edge. On foot, driving their mules, carrying corn as food for mules and man and black beans for man, they slowly worked their way through the jungle country. Every year the distance became greater. In those days mule pack trains returned the accumulated chicle throughout the wet season over these same routes, ending up at narrow-gauge railheads, lake barges, or other collection points. Now and for several past years the problem of distance has been taken out of the chicle jungles. Airplanes bear the chiclero and his supplies to improvised landing fields, which still may be miles away from the chicle camps. In turn these planes transport the collected chicle to railheads or seaports. Around the jungle landing field a few women may be found among the dozen or more men who receive and wrap up the blocks or marquetas of chicle brought in from the camps. Almost never do women go into the camps themselves.

When the rains no longer fall and the sap no longer flows, the camps break up. The chicleros are flown out of the jungle to the season's pay awaiting them and scatter to their numerous pueblos for a five months' respite.

The plane company proved to be as accommodating as the physicians and the photographers. A pretense was made of charging for plane travel, but when the settlement time came at the end of the trips an astonishing bill of only $6.25 was laid before me. The desire is to name this chicle transportation company, but because of happenings on one flight this name must remain undisclosed. The company might be offended.

After many days of preparation the time came for taking off. There I was in a wide sombrero hat, high boots, heavy riding pants, to none of which I was accustomed. When I first saw the plane, which had been brought in for my special transportation — there were no other "pay" passengers — all courage left me. If there had been no skeptical gallery to see me off, then and there the journey would have ended. Very clearly I recognized that I was out of my element, in a primitive land, facing a tiny and decrepit plane with a pilot of dubious flying experience. Never did I so long for my own lares and penates. Heartily I wished that either the pilot or I might have a sudden heart attack, or that the plane might catch fire or collapse. My one hundred and ninety pounds and six feet two seemed completely to fill the makeshift cargo pit, but in fear I shrank to smaller size when I found we were transporting a load of explosive oxyacetylene gases for the purpose of repairing a plane that had crashed on the previous day. In the seatless cabin were two nondescript natives going along to do the welding on the wrecked plane. They proved to be handy a few hours later on our own plane.

All of my preparation might forecast a plane journey of ten thousand miles. Scorning four-flushing, I abandon any such pretense. In the jungle two hundred miles is a long distance — two or even three weeks by mule pack. This was the extent of our journey. In a few hours Carlos, the pilot, who professed to speak no word of English, pointed downward to a little village at the jungle's edge. Then with his finger he indicated our prospective descent there.

I made signs inquiring, "Where is the landing field?"

Carlos pointed to a widened earthen road. One of the native welders who spoke a little English said that a stiff wind was blowing directly across the line of our landing and that the landing would be "rough." Also he translated a remark of the pilot, "my sweetheart is down there and I am thinking of her." This becomes important in the light of what happened one minute later. The maneuver of the pilot in descending was physiologically devastating — he merely corkscrewed.

Having been warned that the landing would be rough, I closed my eyes. Carlos, apart from thinking of his sweetheart, was perhaps only remembering that on that field he usually landed with chicle loads of about four times the rated maximum capacity of the plane. Apparently this was the sort of landing that Carlos scheduled. We touched the ground, then there began a series of crashes, slashes, tears, rents. I, with my eyes still closed, was only thinking, "This is worse than promised." Then all was quiet and I opened my eyes. We were in the tree tops — in truth very small trees; one wing was gone; no landing gear was left, and the propeller blades looked like bent spoons. On our various ups and downs we had gone through the stone wall of a nearby native cemetery, which seemed appropriate.

The pilot, true to his profession, first thought of his passenger and miraculously spoke in English — this for the first time — saying, "Now we are safe. The danger is over."

I, trying to be composed and nonchalant, said, "This is the way I always prefer to land."

Then the pilot passed out — not dead — only fainted.

Soon natives came running from all directions. Knowing that we might be grounded for several days, although prophetically we had transported our repairing welders with us, I sensed a good opportunity to become friendly with these natives, from whom I hoped to learn many things. I pitched in quite manfully in helping prepare a pathway from the so-called landing field out to the wrecked plane. I toted and piled up rocks from the pathway and dragged brush cut by the volunteering Indians with their always-on-hand machetes. Soon I noticed that all of these Indians were close around me, following every move. My scheme was working too successfully. I was attracting too much attention. At that moment there appeared the interpreter sent in for services with me by the sometimes planful aviation company. At once I inquired why all of the native interest in me and not in the wreck. His reply was immediate.

"They think you are a giant. They have never seen anybody as big as you are. They think that maybe your very weight wrecked the plane."

Soon another disturbing event. From the first, a few dogs visited the wreckage. One whiff of me convinced them that never in their canine experience with odors had they encountered my precise variety. This upset their equanimity. Previously they perhaps felt that they had whiffed every known odor. Now all calculations failed. After that wreck, I would not have been surprised at any odor about me. This important development in dog life was bruited over the countryside. Dogs came running from all directions at their highest speeds. They rushed in for one sniff and retired for contemplation. Man and dog, I had a following.

By nearly nightfall all that could be done to the plane save by the welders had been done. My precious baggage had not been harmed. The explosives were intact. We started for the village, a mile away, where I had been promised quarters in a mule stable, the mules being on duty in a chicle camp. The first unit in the parade was one over-sized doctor, convoyed by a milling whirlpool of dogs. The second phalanx was comprised of every man, woman, and child of the village. The rear was brought up by a half-dozen befuddled landing field employees and pilots, concocting the alibis for the wrecks — three in one week.

Life in a stable is not so bad — particularly when you are in a warm state of gratitude over being alive. Of course, it took some readjustment to adapt oneself to the mule water-trough without running water as the supply for bathing, cooking, and for my stable mates' drinking purposes. This was not a one-mule stable. Perhaps designed for six mules, it accommodated some twenty of those of us who were guests of the village, visiting pilots and busy welders.

My friends, the village people, rightly figured that the prospects of my sleeping comfortably in a hammock were not good. A bed was promised — the mayor's — there being two beds in the village. I conceived the arrival of a nice, wide, long, four-poster with a double mattress and built-in springs. What actually arrived was a frame on the top of two "X's" to which was nailed canvas. The entire populace came down for the bed installation, some never having seen a bed. With ostentation, it was placed at my disposal. I hope that I was humble and gracious in accepting it. Some of my stable-mates slept squatting in packing cases, others on the floor, one on a table, and one just squatting. Four days later, when I left the stable, at three o'clock in the morning, as I closed the door a nineteen-man riot broke out in a fight for the use of my bed. I never learned who won.

This village furnished many cases of the disease of my search. The village physician, Dr. Aguilar, brought together, by eight o'clock the next morning, several patients. Long histories were taken, endless questions asked, photographs made, other cases inquired about, treatments observed. Some of the natives crowded into the doctor's office for their own observations.

In the midst of this medical jamboree, in rushed an excited youth, who stated that a woman of the village had in her possession the very fly that had bitten her husband, who in time had acquired the chiclero's disease. It was her prize possession, for which she had been offered considerable money. This fly in that village had certain mystical values, since it was believed that if you looked upon the fly it wouldn't be there. This gets over into something akin to voodoo, which is no part of this narrative. En masse we marched to this lady's house. Her husband was away in some chicle camp, disease and all. Quite respectfully the crowd remained on the outside of the little oval, floorless, thatched hut. Three of us entered, the manager of the chicle assembly activities, the interpreter, and myself. The lady was flattered by so much attention. It was an occasion when the whole village stood in front of her house because of interest in her. Only her funeral would have attracted this throng otherwise, and she perhaps could have gotten no enjoyment out of that.

First my interpreter made a speech in the appropriate dialect in which he apparently drew some longbows, extolling the capacities of scientific endeavor and promising perhaps that the chiclero's disease thenceforth would pass out of existence. This was followed by a melodious speech by the proud owner of the fly, held before her wrapped up in a scrap of newspaper. She pointed out that she would accept under no circumstances any money from the visiting scientist but, because she herself was deeply interested in science, would donate the remarkable fly. You all have seen this very same sort of ceremony go on in the midst of high hats and long coats when wealthy foundations benevolently dedicate great edifices to the cause of science. The scoffers then are wont to make remarks about stuffed shirts; but in Quintana-Roo, in this bare hut, the situation was genuine. In due course it seemed necessary that my word be added to the lot. Through the interpreter, I thanked the benevolent lady for her great gift, praised her for her unwillingness to accept money and expressed the hope that this fly might in fact be found to stand in some causative relation to a disease that beset her people.

Later on, having no knowledge whatever of entomology, I sent this insect to Harvard University for identification, after having hauled it around several thousand miles. Back came the scornful response from Harvard, stating, "This is no fly at all, but a bee. It could not possibly bite and not even remotely could be related to the disease of the chicleros."

That possibly might have been anticipated.

Back at the corral, on another morning, when at last I was left alone by the people, there came the man with the "pink pants." I was very busy boiling my canned beef in a bucket of the horse-trough water. Over my shoulder came a voice, authoritative and positive, "That is not the way to do that. You should dump the beef into the water."

I replied, and I hope equally positively, "But this is the way that I want to do this."

Back came the voice, "Very well, every man has a right to his own particular way of killing a buzzard. If that's your way, go ahead."

I turned and there was the man not only in the pink pants, but in the green shirt — toothless before his day, and in himself an epitome of all that was bizarre in those queer lands — gaunt, angular, bossy, obviously an outlander, and clearly of importance.

The man in the "pink pants" was ready to talk; in fact he gave every evidence of being a man who had not talked in a long time and would fight for the opportunity. Talk at once poured out that lasted all day. He was the "boss chiclero" in a large camp several hundred miles away. That morning he had flown in to pick up a shipment of twine for tying up his marquetas of chicle. Not for nine months had he been out of his camp, nor even seen a piece of money, because in a chicle camp there is no occasion for spending money — nothing to buy, nothing to sell. Money had been sent to him in this village. His chief desire was to return to the knack of spending money. He bought right and left of repulsive candies, fifth-rate bottled pops. We played pool at his expense. He bought a shuck underpad for a horse collar, not because he had any need for such an object, but merely to restore him to the art of spending money. When I inquired why he hadn't left his hammock, which he carried about everywhere with him, with his luggage, he replied, "This is all my luggage."

This, he pointed out, was his only necessity, as constantly with him as the machete is with an Indian. His lack of teeth attested his disbelief in the toothbrush and tooth powder as any part of traveling needs. I, of course, wanted to know about chiclero's ulcer in his camp. He said, "Yes, about sixty per cent of my nine hundred men have chiclero's disease — no — no treatment is ever carried out. No chiclero is ever worth it. The chiclero is worth only three cents in State's money. Why spend money for treatment? They aren't worth it. Besides, nearly all of them die of snakebite. During the last season, three hundred of my nine hundred men died of snakebite. The snake with the 'four noses' bit them. The next day they died. There is no need to try to get them to a doctor, even by plane. It is too far away. Occasionally one lives, but maybe he wasn't bitten very deep."

"How do your men get this chiclero's disease?"

"They seem always to have had it. Some men in my camp say they have had the disease for thirty years. It comes and goes. They never get well, but sometimes they don't get worse."

"What causes the disease?"

"Everybody has a different idea. Some say a big fly, some a little fly, some a green fly, some a black and white fly; some men say they brush against the small underbrush and get the disease. Some say a little tiny mite bites them. Some of the men believe that when the hunters bring in a deer the flies are on the deer and they leave the deer and bite the men. Take your choice, brother. As for me, I don't believe any of it and don't give a damn anyway. I never got the disease."

So I shared my canned pears with the man in the pink pants and took occasion to ask him what his job was before he became a boss chiclero. He replied, "I was a silk buyer in Paris and passed on most of the silks shipped out of France to the United States."

Later that night Carlos, the pilot, who continued to admit that he could speak a little English, took me aside and told me not to pay any attention to the man in the "pink pants," not that that was his term for him.

He said, "Once a year he comes to town to practice talking, just as he has to relearn how to spend money. He probably never had three hundred men in his whole camp. If two of his men died of snakebite last year, that probably would be a record. When he said 'three hundred' he probably was just practicing saying 'three hundred'."

The time came for me to fly into the deep jungle — the same sort of plane, an overload of corn for the mules, my faithful interpreter, but a new pilot. If I thought the landing field at the receiving end of the plane line was bad, I should have anticipated the one at the shipping point. For a while we could not land at all because mules were nibbling on the grass at this one open spot in the thick forest. In time, some of the chicleros drove off the mules at least for a pathway as wide as our plane. I calculated the train of events in case one or more of the mules decided to return to the landing way. Alongside the runway were great piles of chicle in neat bales ready for loading.

A fair number of the chicle gatherers had come in from their remote camps to this loading station. Here was chiclero's disease in epidemic quantities. Here was the end of the journey. Soon the plane that brought us took off with its quadruple load, just clearing the stumps at the end of the runway.

THEN BEGAN endless inquiry, the taking of samples of blood, and the making of photographs. Every step of the work was traced, every detail of camp life, the cutting of the trees, the boiling of the sap, the molding of the marquetas, the bringing in of corn for tortillas. In the midst of these conferences in which the chicleros eagerly and honestly related their stories, in came the hunter with a peccary. That meant meat for supper — for everyone except the finicky visitor. The interpreter had no qualms. Black bean soup, pink chicos, and hurriedly roasted peccary made up the camp banquet. This was washed down by a thin, watery mixture made by sloshing a handful of cornmeal paste in about two gallons of water. By the time of the end of the banquet the notebooks were filled. At sunset the plane came for us. Hopefully, I had it planned that this plane would take no load of chicle, only its two prospective passengers. I misjudged the situation — a little more than the usual overload was piled into the plane. It was necessary that I climb into the cockpit through a front window the size of which would only have permitted the passage of an eight months old baby without touching the window frame. All this seemed quite unimportant, for by this time I knew some of the answers to chiclero's disease.

When all the notes were put together, a story unfolded. No brilliant discoveries, no credit for the disclosure of a new organism — nonetheless, some new findings.

Chiclero's disease, or jungle ulcer, or chiclero's ulcer, is known to be Leishmaniasis, a well-known tropical disease common in portions of Africa, Asia and Mediterranean Europe. Leishman first discovered this disease, but the particular organisms, in the general class of protozoa, closely related to trypanosomes, are called Leishman-Donovan bodies. For reasons unknown, this disease takes on different forms in different portions of the world, and in some instances only the specific organism is the connecting link in varieties of the disease having practically no features in common. In South America, the skin variety of Leishmaniasis is further varied, and is accorded many local names such as forest yaws, uta, espundia, buba, and pianbois.

Many learned investigations have been carried out, seeking a particular insect that may distribute the disease from person to person, to establish any biologic changes in the organism that may take place in the insect body, and further to disclose anything, bird, beast, or plant that may be the natural reservoir. The phlebotemus fly long has been suspected and by some incriminated as the vector of this disease. None of these things is yet proved.

In the case of the chiclero, a set of peculiar circumstances exists that may make the passage of this disease from person to person apparently simple. These circumstances, limited to the chiclero alone, may account for the high incidence of this disease among these industrial workers. These peculiarities definitely are associated with the trade processes of chicle gathering and thus place the disease, when it so arises, in the category of occupational diseases. The chiclero, as he slashes the sapote tree, is continually sprayed with a shower of bark and chips. His face, arms, torso, and chest are bared and are continually being nicked. The abdomen and lower extremities are covered and rarely present jungle ulcer. The nicked skin of the upper portion of the body bleeds a little — a drop here and there. In these camps, small or large, always there are afflicted workers with open ulcers. They are the reservoirs. Likewise, in the jungle there are a great variety of flies, some of which are blood suckers, some merely feed on the discharged blood. Some undoubtedly feed on the open ulcers of the afflicted and next time feed on the minor abrasions of the unafflicted. Thus the organism probably is transferred from the sick to the well. The kettle tenders and the muleteers seldom have their skins broken, seldom are invaded by the disease producing parasite.

It may not be necessary to conceive of elaborate biologic changes in the organism taking place in the fly, such as regularly attend the cycle of the malarial parasite in the mosquito. Having been fed upon and infected by the fly, a few weeks later a tiny ulcer begins at the point of infection and a new case is started — a new nidus of infection is created for perpetuation of the disease for other chicleros in other seasons. In time, nearly all of the chicleros may be involved to some degree.

You may ask, "How may this disease be prevented?" Granting something nebulous in the theory, it appears that augur boring of the sapote tree instead of slashing might both save the tree and prevent the flying abrading chips; the sap will run out just the same. Apparently, the fewer the abrasions on the unafflicted working amid those who are afflicted, the fewer the new cases of Leishmaniasis. If all of the afflicted, through some provision for their livelihood, might be kept out of the jungle and under treatment until cured, it is probable, but not proved, that no new cases would arise within that population.

Within the mechanisms of public health endeavor, this is feasible, and abundant truth-telling results might accrue.

How may this disease be treated? Organic antimonial compounds properly administered will cut short the majority of cases beyond the point of infectivity and within a few weeks, but no new ears may be made to grow. Sometimes treatment fails and recurrences take place. Adequate treatment of all persons afflicted probably would eliminate the reservoirs of infection. Here is a solvable problem in public health.

Economic situations in the countries involved, plus somewhat backward concepts of public health opportunities appear to be the only handicaps to the banishment of this disease as it occurs among the chicleros.

As you bite into a stick of wholesome chewing gum, there is truly nothing effete — no possible connection between any jungle disease and the product you consume. No steps need be taken by any chicle corporation or chewing gum manufacturer better to safeguard your interests as chewing gum consumers in regard to disease transmission. No less, there is a little piece of man in your chewing gum. The chiclero who, with his machete, flies in a crowded plane to the forests of sapote trees in order that you may chew gum contributes a tiny and invisible portion of himself to each of his marquetas. He is little aware of this contribution, and his intellectual level would make difficult any comprehension of his contribution of a little of himself in the product. All work may exact a little toll of the worker, but your servant the chiclero often contributes a generous bit of himself in his effort to please you.

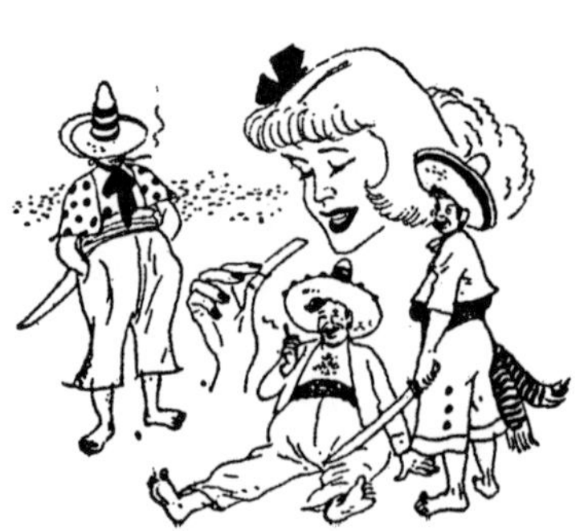

OFT RECCURRING throughout this book is the language "the little piece of man." That McCordism, when the writing is done on the level of feeling and not on the level of the technical, refers to the worker's day by day invisible attrition of body and mind — a little into every unit of his wares. For forty years this concept has occasionally climbed up on the typewriter keys demanding a hearing. It is high time its beginning be disclosed.

Chapter 11

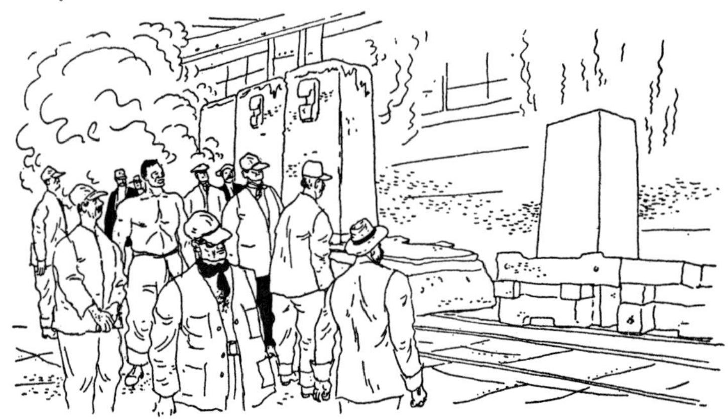

A Little Piece of Man

THE steel mill was subdued that day. Down through the blast furnaces, the Bessemer mills, the soaking pits, the open hearth furnaces, the rolling mills, the sheet mills — everywhere men were subdued. Men walked as with a new load on their shoulders. There was no laughter, no gay waving of arms.

A stony dignity marked all.

At the far end of the plant, on a hummock apart from any steel making operations stood a stella-like, massive, still hot ingot of steel. Near it, but not close because of its heat, had gathered a group of silent, unmoving people. Unaware of distress, I, just arrived, but sensing something unusual as I passed along the plant's roadways, asked in moderate tones which probably seemed raucous to the hushed group, "What's going on here?"

Quite soberly one bystander pointed to the upright ingot, saying, "There's a man in there. Last night one of the ladle men fell into an ingot mold just at the time it was being poured with steel. Of course, he was burnt up. Whatever is left of him is in that ingot. Some of these folks are his family."

I felt I had been a little disrespectful.

Calamity had struck again. A troubled management scarcely knew how to dispose of a steel ingot's many tons that shrouded a worker. His sorrowing family and friends were equally bewildered. It was not thinkable that this ingot might be rolled into steel rails. The victim, had he any choice might have elected to have been transformed into rails. As millions of car miles rolled over his body's elements, possibly a little gaily and proudly he might have sung to the clacking of moving wheels, "I gave much to a nation's progress — to the growth of a land." But this was not done.

It was equally incongruous that this massive ingot might be hauled into any church for a burial ceremony.

In a little time, a considerate and appropriate solution was found. At one end of the plant area, apart from any operations, was a small grove of trees. An improvised quarter mile of railroad track was

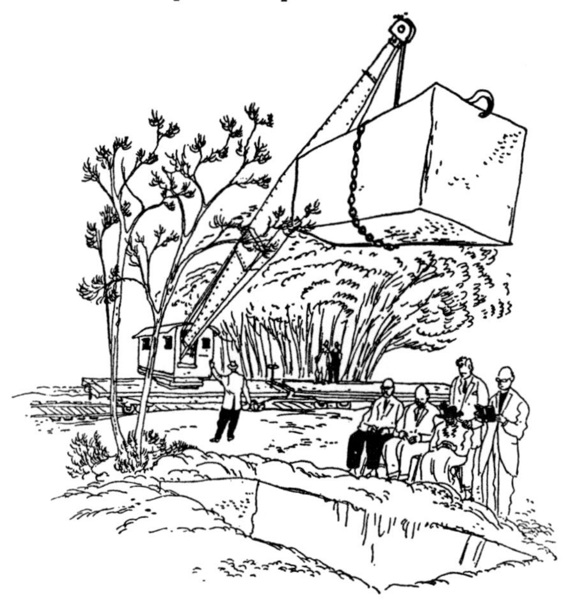

laid down and the railroad crane transported the steel ingot with its human content to that spot. A grave was dug and the entire ingot buried, with services appropriate to the dead man's religious beliefs. Thus ended for the eyesight of man a distressing occurrence.

For me, the awe lasted. Not awe quickly transmuted into action, just awe as awe. The fate of the man possessed me, "There's a man in there. There's a man in there." That was more than forty years ago. Slowly has come the understanding that all products exact a minor toll of their producers. In every made thing about you is a little piece of man. As you hold this book you hold tiny portions of many men and women — the maker of the type, the creator of the printing ink, the producer of the paper, the printer, the proofreader, the binder, and the publisher who worries over the possibilities that this book may not earn its keep.

It is a happy circumstance that all of honest toil takes a little toll — the laudable wear and tear of labor — the beads of excessive perspiration — tasks that make for hearty appetites — stints that assure sleep, sound and undisturbed. This physiologic toll fosters the pride of artisanship in a product's maker—gentle fatigue adds to the satisfaction of labor. But, there is a limit, a threshold of beginning injury and beyond this threshold lies possible havoc.

That's where the industrial hygienist comes in. His job is to keep "man" out of "manufactures."

Chapter 12

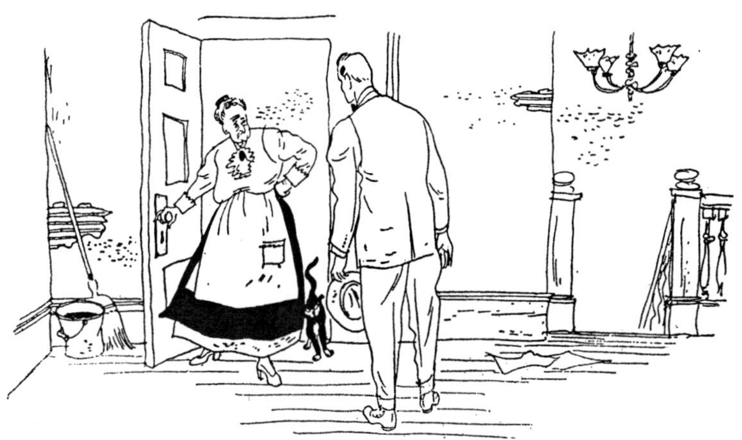

Coroner for a Day

As surely as the cartoonist's saw and log instantly register "snorer" in the public mind, so do beard, stethoscope and head mirror quickly label "doctor." It is something of an anachronism that the physician is still portrayed as bearded, for bearded doctors are as rare as bearded ladies. Moreover, the day of the doctor may hold infinitely more than what he sees through the head mirror or hears through the stethoscope. Long ago, when I was the physician in charge of a department store employee hospital, I demonstrated the perfect antithesis of this popular conception.

The experience really began the first time I saw Addison Grayman who had come into my office for a pre-employment physical examination. Applying for the job of carpenter's assistant, Grayman's card stated that he was twenty-three, unmarried and had no local address because he had just arrived in the city. His nearest relative was his father, Westley Grayman, of Buford, West Virginia. All of this I noted. Grayman got the job.

On the afternoon of his first day of work, the new carpenter's assistant and a crew of workmen were moving long store tables from the basement to the seventh floor. In the procedure the freight elevator was stopped at the sixth floor and the tables hoisted through the opening on the floor above. As the tables emerged, the carpenter's foreman occasionally would yell to the elevator operator, "Hoist." By arrangement, the elevator then would be moved up two or three feet. On one of these "hoists" the new and awkward employee was caught across the abdomen between the end of the table and the nearby wall. Disclaiming any injury, he was nevertheless immediately brought to my office. Indeed, there was no mark of injury, no bruise or scratch on his body. With caution born of experience, I insisted that he be hospitalized for the night, especially since he had no local home. Despite his rebellious protests, he was sent to the hospital in the store's medical car and placed under the observation of an able surgeon. During the night crushing internal injuries that escaped all previous examinations appeared. Addison Grayman died.

The following morning a telegram was sent to the police in Buford, West Virginia:

"PLEASE LOCATE WESTLEY GRAYMAN, FATHER OF ADDISON GRAYMAN OF YOUR TOWN AND ADVISE OF HIS UNFORTUNATE ACCIDENT AND DEATH YESTERDAY. ADVISE IF FATHER AS NEXT OF KIN WILL CLAIM BODY."

Soon came the police reply:

"NO SUCH PARTY KNOWN IN THIS COMMUNITY."

Somewhat more than surprised, I hastened over to the coroner's office, reporting, "We had an accidental death in one of our employees last night. It's clearly a case for you. Will you take over from here?"

Ordinarily the most genial and hearty of men, the coroner lost every trace of good will at my words. With doleful expression and in grieved tones, he replied, "Look at me. Here I am all dressed to start on a hunting trip and you want me to investigate a death." We looked blankly at each other, and suddenly he was inspired.

"Here, take my badge. You be coroner until I get back. Hold the body and we'll have the inquest day after tomorrow, when I return."

With a shrug I accepted the badge, thinking for a moment that the prospect of being coroner might be pleasant. Short-lived was the moment.

The noon edition of the city paper appeared on the street with the headlines:

> "WIFE OF INJURED WORKMAN WALKS STREETS WHILE HUSBAND DIES IN HOSPITAL"
>
> "Addison Grayman, residing at 210 Plymouth Street, died last night in Christian Hospital following injury at Bossman Brothers Department Store. Store management failed to notify this man's family of injury. His wife spent the night walking the streets searching for her husband who had failed to return home at the usual hour. During this period, Grayman died following an emergency operation."

Poor public relations for any store. Here were beginning complications for the coroner of the day. I rushed back to the store to re-examine Addison Grayman's employment card. In the dead workman's own handwriting there still appeared "Unmarried"—nearest of kin, "Father." I looked again at the telegram from Buford. "NO SUCH PARTY KNOWN IN THIS COMMUNITY."

It occurred to me rather strongly that, as coroner, I had been left holding the body. Two-ten Plymouth Street proved to be a rooming house, and a sordid one at that. A fishy-eyed landlady responded to my knock and impassively admitted me.

"Does Mrs. Addison Grayman reside here?" I asked, stepping into the dark hallway. Cabbage and human odors vied with each other for preeminence in the atmosphere.

Mrs. Fishy-Eyes sniffed before answering. "She lives here."

"May I speak with Mrs. Grayman?" I ventured.

She eyed me suspiciously, the glossed, liquid eyeballs covering my length and noting, perhaps, the white collar.

"So you're from that there department store are you?" she exploded suddenly. "So it's the likes of you that lets a poor woman walk the streets all night lookin' for a dead man? Well, the poor soul, God rest her, ain't come back yet, and you'll like to have her on your conscience too, her probably being at this minit worn out and taken to some hospital."

"You've not seen her?" I asked quietly.

"No, I've not seen her — not since she rushed out into the street in her grief, sobbing and crying like a mad woman, and I don't blame her, as who wouldn't."

"Well," I said, bringing forth my coroner's badge, "as coroner I'd like to examine the dead man's room, if you'll lead the way."

However unworthily worn, the badge had the desired effect, and I was taken to Grayman's room. Nothing there aided the situation. Everything was feminine but one suitcase which contained a few articles of male clothing and several letters. These were from Pittsburgh, Buffalo, Reading, and Wheeling. All were from men and chiefly indicated the opinion that no work was to be had in those cities. The landlady had accompanied me and stood interestedly by while I made the examination. She continued to rant against Bossman Brothers, but managed to exclude me from more than a minor share of guilt.

"It's really too bad I can't locate Mrs. Grayman," I said casually as we walked downstairs. "She's entitled to six thousand dollars compensation and funeral expenses."

"Six thousand dollars?" she repeated, brightening visibly.

"Yes," I assured her, "and the Industrial Commission Board pays the funeral expenses."

Reaching the door, she said, "Well, maybe I can locate the widow — poor, grieving soul."

Not much more than an hour later the elusive Mrs. Grayman appeared in the coroner's office, seeming little in need of consolation. Her first question was illuminating.

"Is it true I get six thousand dollars as a widow's award?" She spoke quickly, her demeanor greedy rather than grieving.

"Yes, madam," I replied. "If you are his widow and dependent the normal death award for an industrial accident is six thousand dollars in this state."

"Poor Addison," she murmured with downcast eyes.

"Will you claim the body after the inquest and make burial arrangements?" I asked.

"Certainly I shall take care of funeral arrangements," she promised, and left quickly.

I continued to wonder about that "Unmarried" on the employment card, that and the practical-minded little widow. Interrupting my train of thought came an excited reporter.

"We've just had a long distance call from Dayton and some guy claims he's Addison Grayman!"

"Say that again," I exclaimed.

"Yeah, you heard right. This guy's claiming he's Grayman and that his wife lives at 210 Plymouth Street, and he's not dead."

"He's sure of that, I presume. . . ."

"He wants an immediate retraction and he's coming on to find out what this is all about."

Admittedly, I was a little curious on that score myself and a bit resentful thinking of the real coroner killing ducks while we had a corpse come to life, disturbingly. Soon the widow returned, outwardly a widow. She was sheathed in black from head to foot, even carrying a black bordered handkerchief. The amateur coroner decided to throw a trial bombshell.

Softly I said, "Your Dayton husband is on his way down."

A direct hit resulted. She jumped to her feet in panic and began edging toward the door. I blocked her passage. "Now tell me the real truth," I said angrily.

Cringing, fright-stricken, the sordid soul poured out her more sordid story. "This dead man ain't my husband. I picked him up on the street two days ago. He had no money and no home. My landlady knew I had a husband, but she ain't never seen him so I took this guy home and let him use my husband's name. He used it when he got that job at Bossmans."

"What is the real name of the dead man?" I demanded.

"Baker, Harry Baker. Look what he's done to me now — gettin' killed, and all I've done for him."

"Most ungrateful of him," I remarked dryly.

"Yeah, and I'm gettin' out before Grayman gets here. He'll never find me."

Feeling sure the real Addison Grayman would survive the loss of an encounter with his wife, I permitted the erstwhile mourner to leave. She apparently went far away — and fast. A blustering toolmaker established his living and the right to the name in question, and the episode of Addison was ended.

Another and more fitting telegram was sent to Buford where Harry Baker's sorrowing and shamed old mother and father claimed responsibility for their wayward son, wondering, perhaps, over the evils of a world in which in their simplicity they played no understanding parts.

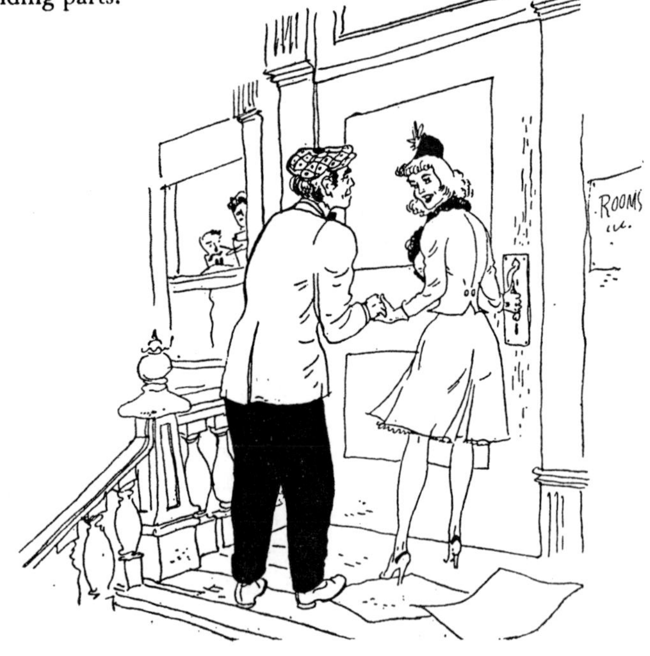

Chapter 13

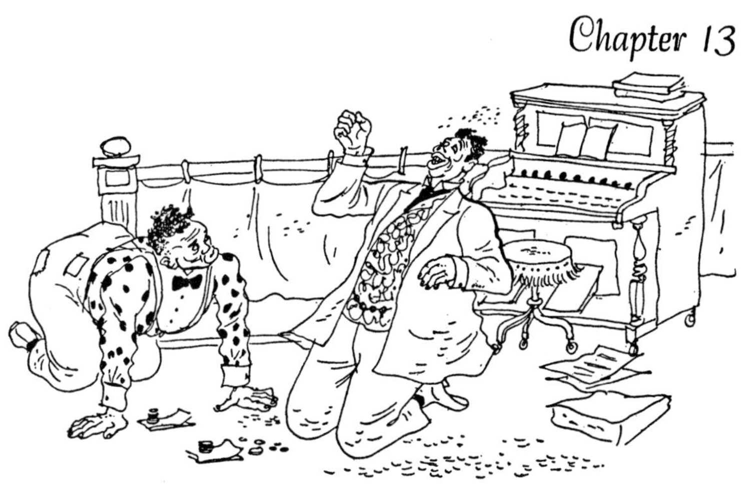

Panic

THE HUMAN mind, marvel that it is even in its lowest example, is far from perfect.

In and out of industry, the usually rational individual mind and the minds of entire groups, on rare occasion temporarily wholly desert their owners. These little minds, no longer there, take with them all proper responses to what their eyes see or their ears hear. Unfortunately, the faculty of speech and screaming are left behind for insane use.

The round of tasks for all industrial hygienists, myself included, is sprinkled with episodes of feckless mental routs — individual hysteria, mass hysteria, panic. The toxic agent is no gas, dust, or vapor from some industrially used chemical; instead, it is the mischievous contrivance of a mind or minds suddenly cut loose from stability. One distinguished American industrial hygienist, in describing such a sorry happening in Russia, records that only in Russia might such a disaster take place. Sadly enough, right here in the

United States worker groups and other groups are susceptible—very, very vulnerable.

My first encounter long antedates any personal medical appraisal, when I was a late arrival at the scene of one of the country's most foolish disasters.

In one Alabama city a negro religious denomination was assembled in a week-long statewide convention. Its sessions were held in a shabby auditorium seating many hundreds of persons. At one night's session, the choir in its loft had carried out its pre-address function and settled down to long winded orations by speakers on the platform below. Two of the singers, essaying to while away the tedious moments until their vocal talents next might be needed, were indulging in the pastime of crap rolling on the carpeted loft floor, well hidden by the thigh-high curtains in front. The shooting of the dice apparently did not progress to the satisfaction of one of the two, so that then and there was started a none too Christian-like pummeling. This form of settling difficulties reached such a state of rolling bodies and flailing arms as to come into the view of some of the brethren seated in the balcony. One, lusty-lunged, and perhaps more excited over the choir loft happenings than those about the dais below, yelled "Fight, Fight." Building acoustics played a mean trick on the multitude. "Fight, Fight" was tranformed into "Fire, Fire." Within the duration of a breath, the crowd was turned into a seething mob, milling, pushing, shoving, trampling of bodies, breaking of windows; men, women and children were caught between torn-up pews. As ever, the overflow crowd on the outside, hearing the tumult, in curiosity tried to force their way inward. Some devotees, in complete mental rout, jumped from balcony level windows and were killed. Within twenty minutes there were scores of torn, maimed, broken bodies. If long memory actually serves, there were near a hundred and forty deaths. The exact number is a matter of record in that city's annals of tragedy.

Through endless variation and without provocation such events unhappily occur in industry and more often among women.

In my office sat a young married worker with a minor but obscure skin disease. I did not know its nature and frankly told her so. Quite casually I remarked, "If you were pregnant I probably could make a diagnosis."

She was not pregnant, but the idea gripped her. "I didn't know I was pregnant," she exclaimed beaming. "I was even examined by my family doctor. Why didn't he know I was pregnant?"

"But, Madam, you misunderstood. I did not say you ARE, I said IF."

"I'm so glad," she interrupted. "Oh, I'm so glad. Max and I have wanted a baby for so long." Her voice was confidential. "I am glad."

"No. No. No." I said leading forward. . . .

"A baby," she murmured dreamily.

"No," I said again jumping to my feet. "No, Madam — I merely remarked. . . ."

"How long may I work?" she asked. "Can I go on working now that I'm pregnant?"

In complete exasperation I left the room to cool off. When I returned she got in the first words. "I've been thinking that since you were the first to tell me about the baby, we could name him for you," she smiled upon me.

"Please, Lady," I pleaded. "Let me talk. You are not pregnant. Certainly I have no idea that you are pregnant."

"Max will want a boy," she said blandly.

Wincing, I continued, "Your skin disease is the type that sometimes shows up in pregnant women." I spoke slowly and carefully. "Whatever it is, it's quite simple. You don't have to bother quitting. Go on and work."

"You know," she confided, "I don't really care whether it's a boy or girl." Her hands went through the motions of knitting tiny garments as she sat. My words had fallen on completely blocked off ears. In desperation I eased her out of the office and watched her depart in a shining aura of maternity, walking stiltedly to protect her unborn infant.

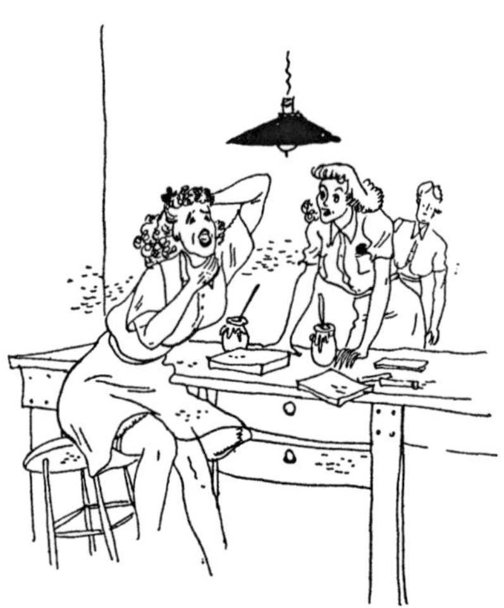

However well the latter case portrays mental blocking in the case of the individual, it fails to picture the utter rout that seizes groups of people, the panic of every individual exalting the same state in every other.

One May morning, at the Caldwell Texler Novelty Company, some eighty women were working on the second floor making minor wood and cardboard assemblies, using no more deadly material about them than small quantities of ordinary wood glue. One girl looked up suddenly and announced above the low conversational murmur, "I smell something." Others stopped working to sniff. "It's burning my eyes," she shouted, then clutching her throat she screamed, "It's choking me! It's poisoning me!" Off her chair down to the floor she dropped. Immediately a second woman felt the same symptoms. "I can't breathe," she croaked, falling prostrate beside the first victim. A minute later several other women were unable to breath, victims of something they could not see.

Panic exploded. Down fell woman after woman, retching, vomiting, tearing clothing, rolling on the floor, upsetting equipment, screaming wildly. Fear was tossed about the work room like a ray of light in the hall of a thousand angular mirrors. Within ten minutes fifty women were prostrate. Others trampled one another in flight to safety. Attempts to rescue the afflicted were made by a few. Emergency help rushed from all quarters of the plant.

Doctors, ambulances, life-saving squads, fire department, police department, factory inspection department, public health department and reporters were quickly on the scene. Men dashed into the plant with litters. In mad panic two legs were broken, a dozen ankles sprained, elbows bruised, heads battered. Women shrieked continuously. Trucks were pressed into service, and hospital receiving rooms jammed. Soon strident headlines alarmed the city.

I participated in this havoc, only from what probably best should be termed "an uncontrol tower"— at least a remote post of comparative calm.

One hospital called stating, "We've got a lot of these women from the Caldwell plant on our hands, and we think that it's probably due to cyanide. How do we test to make sure."

I suggested the possibilities and they rushed into action.

Soon another hospital laboratory chief 'phoned in, "We have about a dozen of these women that have been gassed and we suspect nitrogen gases. How do we prove it?"

I suggested the possibilities.

In a little while a third call, expressing the belief that hydrogen sulfide had caused the trouble and asking for aid, was received. Apparently, hospitals had caught the disease.

When the last victim had been removed to safety and pandemonium gave way to a semblance of sanity, proper investigations began. It was found that a janitor had been cleaning out the furnace. But there had been no fire in the furnace for two weeks. Carbon monoxide was ruled out. An insect exterminator some weeks before had applied hydrocyanic gas in a remote portion of the building and had left behind some harmless equipment — nothing that would have generated gas. This possibility was eliminated. One glue pot had boiled over in the early morning and had provided some minor odors of burnt glue. This was about as dangerous as the odors from one unwashed human body.

All of the possibilities were investigated.

By this time some of the victims were being discharged by the hospitals and a little sheepishly they returned to their work benches. In time, the solid truth came to the fore. It was springtime and a few windows had been opened. The plant was located at a busy street intersection. Dozens of automobiles were discharging spent odoriferous exhausts. A trace had drifted into the plant. No greater quantity than attacks the nostrils at any busy street crossing — merely the odors from a little burned oil. This was the monster.

Compensation boards, like the Lord, move in mysterious ways their wonders to perform. A few real injuries, some of which occurred in flight off the plant premises, all were judged to represent accidents arising in the normal course of work. Due compensation and medical bills were paid.

Here's no expressed desire to joust with those who legally dispense the manufacturers' dollars to those duly injured at work. But "Please, Misters and Mesdames, shouldn't that word 'normal' have been left out of a record of reality?"

The runner-up for the fury of the women scorned is that other fury of groups of women caught redhanded in mass panic in the absence of any iota of substantial cause.

If you are a brave man, caring not for the intactness of flesh and bone, or if you doubt the fury that lies buried in the bosoms of women who half-naked have rolled on the floor in stark ridiculousness over nothing, then just step into that department on the second floor and innocently inquire, "Ladies, how is the gas situation today?"

Chapter 14

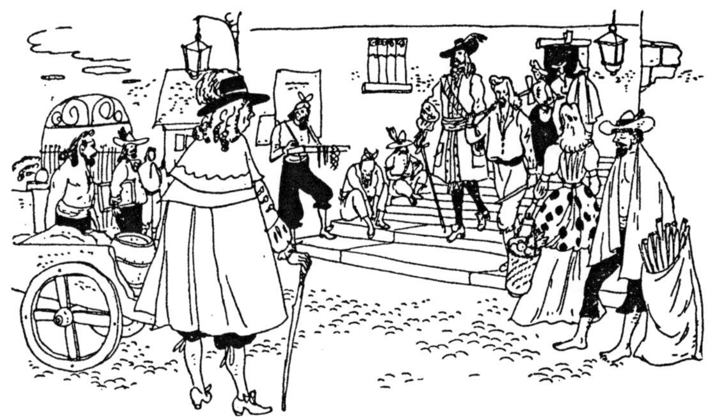

My Boss

MY NEIGHBOR down the road, a man given to many conferences, once confided: "Doctor, when I am with strangers and things are getting a little bumfuzzled, I am apt to say to the group, 'Gentlemen, don't you think all this is quite incongruvial?'

"Of course, Doctor," he ambled on, "There is no such word as 'incongruvial' but its use will cut a verbal gallop to a walk. By the time their tongues are unparalyzed I've had time to pull my own bumble-dom together. If they look at me reprovingly, I'm apt to say apologetically, 'I think maybe I misspoke myself.' That throws them again."

My own system for gaining time is different, at least when at my own offices — my little ergotocracy. On the wall to the right of my desk is a picture of a distinguished, bewigged old gentleman. When the need comes for a quick diversion — a hasty retreat — it's so easy for me to refer to the picture and say, "That's my boss,"

Always that throws a little tanglefoot into things headed in the wrong direction. Comment flies:

"Doctors have no bosses."

"Mean looking fellow for a boss."

"Why don't you buy him a haircut?"

"Looks like he was diked out to go to a costume ball."

By that moment, the tension is over — sometimes.

The picture, however, serves a more admirable end than derailer of the furies. He is my boss.

Some few persons envy or profess to envy the state of the physician. Pressed for a reason, often given is "You don't have a boss." This not always true assertion may constitute a tragedy.

Everybody, at least at times, needs a boss. A wailing wall seldom may be commendable, but an abridgement in the form of a wailing post may come in mighty handy — even for a physician. I have had a few real bosses — genial and provocative public health officers, smoothly steering deans of colleges, captains of industry. Having prospered under the challenging benevolence of these leaders as bosses I long ago adopted another — Bernadin Ramazzini. You too will profit by the acquaintance with my boss now shared with you.

Two hundred fifty years ago and thereabouts there lived in Italy a remarkable investigator of occupational diseases, who was without the stimulus of any professional antecedents within a period of centuries and, notwithstanding his abilities as a teacher, no early successors.

From no easy chair did this industrial hygienist predict the coming of a period of occupational diseases and ills of industry. Instead, he lived among the workers, detecting their occupational disease ills, ferreting out precise causes, and creating means of prevention. Without scorn of the modern physician, in truth it may be said of this sire that his grasp of the needs and opportunities of industrial medicine exceeded that of ninety-five per cent of the physicians of today.

With full understanding of his function, this man might justly walk into any official Bureau of Industrial Hygiene of the present time and say, "I take over." This man was Bernardin Ramazzini.

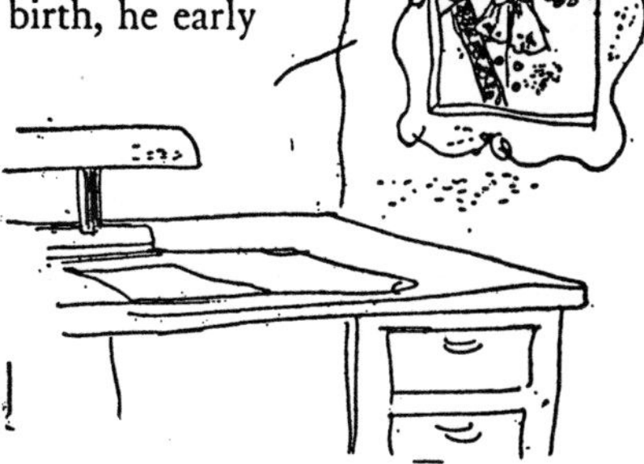

Born in Capri in 1633, he graduated in medicine in Parma in 1659. Returning to Modena, near the place of his birth, he early qualified as a genius by being discredited and maligned by his professional colleagues. This seems to be essential to greatness. Smarting under the barbs of his confreres, he spent much time among the more sympathetic craftsmen of his community. He studied the work of glass makers, painters, dyers, tanners, bakers, millers, stone masons, silk workers, wrestlers, musicians, nurses, porters, grooms, among scores of other trades.

As he went about the business of examining workers, he was not content to ask of the patient, "What uneasiness do you suffer? What was the cause of it? How many days have you been ill? How does your belly stand? What food have you eaten?" But also, and here is what marks him as the sire, "Of what trade are you?"

By 1700, much experience led to his famous book, "De Morbis Artificum Diatriba," (The Diseases of Artificers) — the early gospel of the industrial hygienist.

In this he noted among many hundreds of other observations that potters daubed molten lead over their vessels before placing them in the furnace, thus to produce a glaze. They thus received by "Mouth and Nostrils the Lead Particles and are ceased with Heavy Disorders. Their Hands begin to shake and tremble, soon become Paralytick, Lethargick, Splenetick, Cachectick and Toothless and in time you will scarce see a Potter who has not a leadened death-like Complexion."

Further along in this book he wrote,

> "'Tis well known that dismal Plagues are reflected by Quicksilver upon Goldsmiths and chiefly those who are employed in gilding Silver or Brasswork. For as this Gilding can't be performed without Amalgamation (i.e., the Corrosion of the Metal by Mercury) so when they afterwards come to dislodge this Mercury by Fire, tho they turn away their faces, they can't possibly avoid the receiving of some poysonous Steams at the Mouth, and accordingly we find that this sort of Workmen do quickly become Asthmatick, Paralytick and liable to Vertigo's; and their complexion assumes a dangerous Ghostly Aspect. Few such workmen continue in that way to old Age: or if they do not die betimes, their Condition becomes so miserable, that Death is all their wishes. Their Neck and Hands tremble; their Teeth fall out, their Legs are weak and Maul'd with the Scurvy."

In another chapter of this work, some comment is made upon the occupational diseases of those in preferred professions. Ramazzini, two hundred forty years ago, did a good job in describing the artists of his day. He writes,

> "Painters are also usually subject to various Disorders, such as the Tremblings of the Joynts, a Gachexy, a Blackness of the Teeth, a discolour'd Complexion, Melancholy and loss of Smelling; For it seldom happens that the painters who use to draw the Pictures of others handsome or well Complexion'd than the Originals, are themselves either handsome or well Complexion'd. For my part I have always observ'd that all the Painters I know either in this or other Towns are a'most always sickly; and if we consult the histories of Painters, we'll find they were not long-liv'd; especially if we confine our view to such as made a distinguishing Figure. History informs us that Raphael Urbinus, a very famous Painter, was snatch'd away in the very Flower of his Age; and Balthasar Castiloneus condol'd his untimely Death in a very pretty Poem. 'Tis true, the Diseases of this sort of men may be imputed to their sedentary Life, and the Melancholy that feed upon 'em, while they retire from human Society and bend all their thoughts upon their Phantastick Ideas. But the principal Cause of their Sicklyness is the Matter of the Colours that's always among their Hands, and under their Nose; I mean the Red Lead, Cinnabar, Ceruss, Varnish, Oil of Wallnuts, and Oil of Linseed, with which they temper their Colours, and several other Paints made of various Minerals. Hence 'tis that their Shops have such a nasty stinking Smell, which is chiefly owing to the varnish and foresaid Oils, and is very offensive to the Head; and perhaps the loss of Smell usual

> among Painters flows from no other Cause. Besides, when the Painters are about their work, they have nasty daub'd Cloaths upon 'em, that they can't avoid taking in at Mouth and Nostrils the offensive Exhalations; which, by invading the Seat of the Animal Spirits, and accompanying the Spirits to the blood, disturb the economy of the natural Functions, and give rise to the above mention'd Disorders."

In this country, there are those who regard silicosis, our presently most engaging occupational disease, as something new, peculiar to our own generation. These moderns, unfamiliar with history, turn to LeRoy Gardner, the Chief Investigator of the disease as seen today, as the beginning as well as the end of information on this pneumoconiosis. The more knowing Gardner likely would call attention to Ramazzini's familiarity with this disease of stone hewers, stone cutters, and statue carvers. Ramazzini points out that these workers

> "often times suck in by inspiration, the sharp, rough and corner'd small Splinters of Particles that fly off; so that they are usually troubled with a cough, and some of 'em turn Asthmatick and Consumptive. And in dissecting Corps of such Artificers the Lungs have been found stuffed with little Stones, Diemerbrock gives a curious relation of several Stonecutters that dy'd Asthmatick and were open'd by him; in whose lungs he found such heaps of Sand, that in running the Knife thro' the pulmonary Vesicles, he thought he was cutting some Sandy Body. He adds, that he was inform'd by a Master Stone-cutter, that in cutting Stones there rises such a subtile Dust, as is able to penetrate thro' Ox Bladders hung in the Shop, insomuch that in the space of one Year he found a handful of that Dust in the Cavity of the Bladder; and this very Dust he took to be the cause of the Death of many unwary Workmen."

Though forced into fame by the malice of his colleagues, Ramazzini's genius ultimately was recognized by the Senate of Venice, who made of him the Professor of Medicine at the University of Padua when he was sixty-seven years of age. It was during this period that he published his "Diseases of Artificers" already mentioned. A portion of the front page bears this language:

> "Showing the various influences of particular trades upon the state of health; with the best methods to avoid or correct it; and useful hints

proper to be minded in regulating the cure of diseases incident to tradesmen."

Albeit, in those days, medical books were reserved for the learned professions, this particular one on occupational disease "sold like hotcakes" among the laity, the craftsmen, and among guild members as a guide to their salvation against the wreckage of their trades. It is to be hoped that this note attracts the attention of the present publisher, who possibly may be beguiled into believing that fifty-five million American workmen and eight hundred thousand employers may find my book equally indispensable.

On November 5, 1714, on his eighty-first birthday, while going about his duties at his University in Padua, Ramazzini was stricken with a ruptured blood vessel of the brain and died.

Industrial workers the world over, cannot but cherish the memory of this physician who broke through the conventions and strait-jackets of the centuries and thought it no indignity to learn from scavengers and potters.

Thomas Legge, who has written in admiration and affection of this sire of industrial hygiene, inquires, "What could be a better motto for any manufacturer to lay to heart than the sentence with which Ramazzini closes one chapter of his book?

"'Tis a sordid Profit that's accompany'd with the Destruction of Health."

Devotion to Ramazzini is tenanted by legions. This is attested in the Americas by the "Ramazzini Society." This Society — the servants of Ramazzini — made up of thirty-one physicians whose professional duties center about occupational disease, indulges in only two articles of selfishness: there are no women members, and there are others, over the land, non-members who are qualified by attainments and devotion — their time will come. In the Ramazzini Society there is no place for personal ambitions, for there are no offices or officers, no scientific programs, no by-laws, no funds to be disbursed. But be not misled by any somber implications. Ramaz zini himself long ago set a running pace — far from the somber

Since the Ramazzini Society itself likely would be last to indulge in any flaunting except as homage to the patron saint, and since that society possesses no constitutional niceties through which one recalcitrant member may be disciplined for taking liberties, its small membership soon shall be listed. The reason therefor embodies a little guile. This mild record is highly attenuated autobiography. It needs the roll of some of the fellow travellers.

Dr. Joseph Charles Aub, Boston, Massachusetts.
Dr. E. L. Belknap, Milwaukee, Wisconsin.
Dr. A. G. Cranch, New York, New York.
Dr. J. G. Cunningham, Toronto, Ontario, Canada.
Dr. Cecil K. Drinker, Boston, Massachusetts.
Dr. John H. Foulger, Wilmington, Delaware.
Dr. LeRoy U. Gardner, Saranac Lake, New York.
Dr. Albert S. Gray, Hartford, Connecticut.
Dr. Emery R. Hayhurst, Columbus, Ohio.
Dr. Rutherford T. Johnstone, Los Angeles, California.
Dr. Robert A. Kehoe, Cincinnati, Ohio.
Colonel A. J. Lanza, New York, New York.
Dr. Robert T. Legge, Berkeley, California.
Dr. Christopher Leggo, Oak Ridge, Tennessee.
Colonel Willard F. Machle, Fort Knox, Kentucky.
Commander William S. McCann, Rochester, New York.
Lieutenant Colonel William J. McConnell, Chicago, Illinois.
Dr. William D. McNally, Chicago, Illinois.
Dr. Stuart F. Meek, Detroit, Michigan.
Dr. Paul A. Neal, Bethesda, Maryland.
Dr. Carl M. Peterson, Chicago, Illinois.
Dr. Andrew R. Riddell, Toronto, Ontario, Canada.
Dr. Oscar A. Sander, Milwaukee, Wisconsin.
Dr. C. O. Sappington, Chicago, Illinois.
Dr. R. R. Sayers, Washington, D. C.
Colonel Louis Schwartz, Bethesda, Maryland.
Dr. Clarence D. Selby, Detroit, Michigan.
Dr. Henry F. Smyth, Philadelphia, Pennsylvania.
Dr. James H. Sterner, Rochester, New York.
Dr. W. F. von Oettingen, Bethesda, Maryland.

There is just one drawback to having such a boss or being a Ramazzinian. Stouthearted old Ramazzini was an habitué to "posca," the most villainous of drinks — diluted vinegar — morning, noon, and night —"posca." No devotee may do less than follow the example of the mighty preceptor — but that's hard on the continuity of affections.

Let a plea be made. If anywhere on earth there be any person who two hundred years from now will be the patron saint of anything or anybodies, please, please, sir or madam, engage in no habits of drink which will require that your faithful followers be duty bound to do you homage through gullet-searing "posca."

Chapter 15

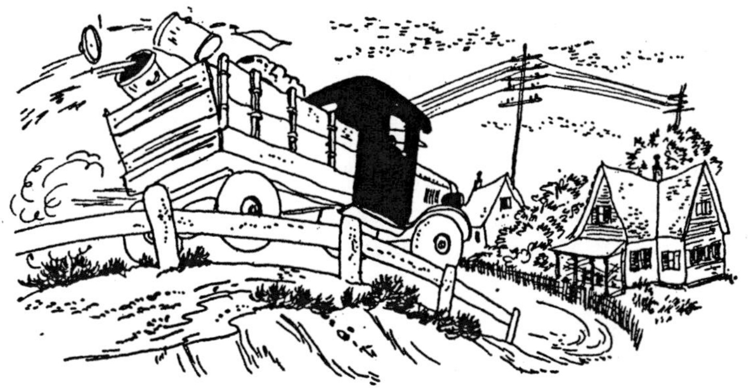

The Offensive Trades

THE ancestry of some of the most treasured, alluring, and seductive of man-made materials is entitled to the merciful protection of a thoroughly beclouding conspiracy of silence.

Some of the most useful and common objects about us, pure and wholesome, have older relatives seldom mentioned other than in the ranks of the immediate family. This is reflected but not condemned in the results of a minor contest among the pupils of a primary school. Everyone was asked to name the thing about them that seemed cleanest and purest. Among others, one named the inside of a cocoanut (which gets my vote for the first prize); another the clean sheets of a newly-made bed; a third a new cake of soap. The soap entry won acclaim, but some soaps and, perhaps, some of the best, shudder over their forebears.

All these implications have to do with a sizable group of honorable and wholly necessary trades harried in modern times by lusty complaints from esthetically disturbed communities.

Do not anticipate any belaboring here of these already hectored manufacturers of these highly essential wares. At all times my sympathies are with them. Their usual background history begets sympathy. In days long ago these plants commonly sought out remote sites, far from the sensitive nostrils and eyes of the emotionally unstable. With increasing populations there came surrounding homes, stores, filling stations, and, in time, also came complaints, injunctions, suits, and trials. Always the manufacturer shouts, "I got here first." He erred in not buying all lands for two miles in all directions.

My guardian angel, in the midst of the writing of this chapter, and verily so, furnished a perfect example of uproarious perturbation incident to an offensive trade.

Near to me a truck well loaded with the offal from a hundred butchered animals, on its way to a plant processing such effete organs, unhappily struck the guarding post of a safety island. In a twinkling, a busy street was flooded with something less pleasing than orchids. Only an anatomist might accept this scene as no less beautiful than a flower show. The policeman assigned to preside over this stew was the most unproud individual viewed in a long while.

But I ask you, "If you scorn entrails, what are you going to do for those life-saving sutures when on the operating table the surgeon is ready to sew up your gaping abdominal wall after his neat repair of your own perforated intestine?"

The English, with their penchant for trade names that fit the case, use a terminology that will make clear at least some of the offensive trades. Without any desire to bring about any twitching of the stomach and solely faithful to reality, a few are here adopted: "fellmongering, blood boiling, gut cleaning, tripe boiling, knacking, manure manufacturing, slaughtering." A little more polite in this country, we lean toward "abattoirs, packing houses, fat rendering, skiving, tankage reduction." A nostril-offended hysterical woman on the witness stand, on referring to the effluvium of the lower of some of these industries, however lexicographically dainty otherwise, is prone to descend to "stinks."

More than one word of disapprobation applied far removed from its origin derives from the offensive trades. A littered hotel room may be described as "in shambles." We really don't mean that. A "shamble" is a slaughter-house.

The badge of the offensive trades is on me.

Over many years, on many occasions, and in several states, I have participated in the abatement of disturbing odors. Since this book runs little to the technical and more to the human happenings in industry, three close-to-the-nose episodes bespeak your tolerance.

ON A DAY in August (the month is important) there came to the laboratory a gentleman "shouting" trouble even before he spoke. He might have been a merchant, a mechanic, or a musician. He wasn't. He was the head of the private garbage-collecting company in his city. Here's his burden:

"Two weeks ago one of our five-ton trucks well loaded with collected garbage was coming down the steep hill on Portia Street. Something went wrong with the brakes. The truck got out of control. At the bottom of the hill the road turns sharply to the left. Straight ahead of the road down the hill is a frame house close up to the street. The driver, seeing he couldn't make the turn, jumped — hoping for a little luck. Maybe we were lucky. At that house a man and his family of four were just sitting down to a meal on the screened-in porch right up near the sidewalk line. That spinning truck was just malicious enough to hit the curb sideways, turn over, break through the screening and slather all those five people, table, chairs, food, with five tons of shall we say, 'not redolent' garbage?"

"From then on . . ." places no burden on the imagination. Heaven save all mankind from the wrath of a woman embedded in garbage.

"Nobody was killed, — but."

"No broken bones, — but."

"That woman is the mother of all the harpies."

"You don't have to be told they are suing us. No objection to replacing the screens or the posts or the floor. Perfectly willing to buy new chairs and a table and dishes. Glad to get them new clothes and all that. What we dislike is that she is claiming she can't get the odors off her body and hair; can't stand the sight of her own garbage pail now; can't do any cooking. She thinks her health is ruined for good. That's where you come in, Doctor. We hope you will help us. We know and you know odors do not injure health. Will you be our witness?"

Then and there I may have uttered my sagest advice. Said I, "I will not be a witness; but you do need a little testimony — right now and from me. Shun a trial on this case as you would a whole peck of hyenas. After all, you can stand only so much jibing. Instead, go right down to the damaged house. See the harpy and her husband. Take your hat off. Be pretty. Be humble. Say in your best manner and with your most ingratiating gesture, 'What is the total damage?' Then take out your check book and your fountain pen and write a check if the amount is anywhere near reason. Take your release and go away from there."

And so he did. Even as he left me he walked not in sorrow but in elation. He knew and I knew that no woman engulfed to the neck in considerably neglected public garbage and at her own dinner table, could ever lose in a court room.

LEAPING across a half dozen states and across twice as many years, we are in sight of a highly modern plant in the offensive trades. The forerunner of this plant had been rural. Its successor on the same site was amid a congested suburban population.

Times ago there may have been grounds for protest; I don't know; I wasn't there. By the time of my arrival already it was nearly modern. I added little. Still there were complaints — mostly imaginary ones. I rushed about the cityside with odorimeters trying to get even a tiny whiff. Always I was met by the belligerents with, "You should have been here just thirty minutes ago. Then there was plenty."

Feeling a little persecuted, we decided to give a party, a friendly neighborhood party, at the plant. We didn't go so far as to plan ice cream and cookies off the trimming tables — at that, we might have. We asked the public to come at a fixed hour of an evening to see the odor quelling machinery, the ozonizers, the chlorination towers, the refrigeration rooms, the water curtains, the condensers. Many accepted. By arrangement we met at a parking lot two blocks away. Mostly by self appointment, I was in charge up to the plant entry. We sauntered along, I fully confident, having found the plant above reproach just one-half hour before. But the crowd was squeamish, uncertain.

A block from the plant and all was serene — then there came an odor as starkly assertive as a bolt of lightning. It rocked me on my heels. It rocked everybody. I reasoned perturbedly, "This is no rendering odor. I know them all." My following did not stay to reason; they fled. So did I.

Not till next morning did the cause of our flight come to light. In that plant were huge bins of stored dried flesh meal widely used for the protein foods of many domestic animals. At the very moment when everything else was putting its best foot forward, some devil of meddlesome design contrived that spontaneous combustion should set up in one meal bin. Perhaps unseen, this had been smouldering for days, until diabolically, at the moment of our coming, it burst loose in odoriferous profusion.

Somewhere there are people who once believed me when I said, "there will be no odors."

Somewhere there are people who trusted me when I argued, "Come and see for yourself. That plant is cleaner than most kitchens."

They see me and cross to the far side of the street. In imagination I hear them saying, "That is the man who tried to fool us on the odors."

As for me, I have learned the great lesson:

Nothing is more linked with imminent disaster than a well meant public demonstration of scientific achievement.

FURTHER travel through time and space ends at a wedding reception. The big house is filled with gay people, champagne, roses, gowns, jewels — out of town guests. The knowing ones are saying, "Of all nights, wouldn't it be dreadful if the stenches broke loose."

The stenches did break loose. Those of the neighborhood knew what was ahead. Astonished women grasped their noses and rushed to powder rooms, wine lost its savor, a few decided then and there they had completed their obligations to the bride and off they went, the cake was uncut, the bride cried, wives looked at husbands reprovingly implying, "If you men had put up a fight sooner, this wouldn't have happened."

Goaded, the fight did come — court action with decorum in the courtroom but hisses in the hallways. The all-wise judge at the proper time ruled, "This complaint has been made only on the grounds of generalities. No particular day or days have been mentioned. This complaint is dismissed for want of a specified time or date."

Disappointment, but not for the defense — for them, jubilation. More indignation. Meetings. Foolish hot heads threatened to bomb the offending plant. Cooler heads chided such foolish ones. A plan was made.

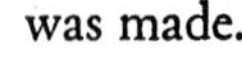

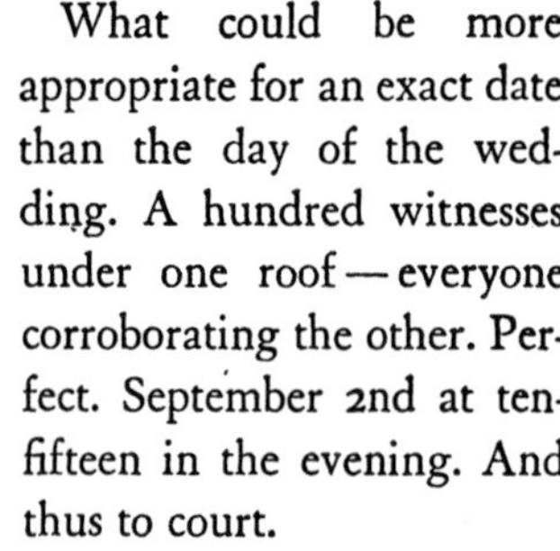

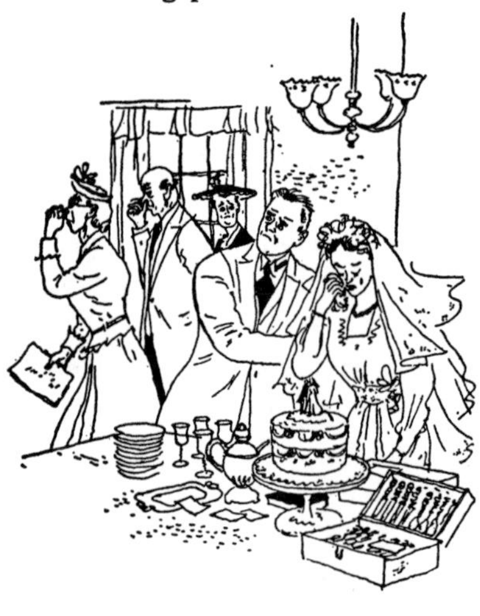

What could be more appropriate for an exact date than the day of the wedding. A hundred witnesses under one roof — everyone corroborating the other. Perfect. September 2nd at ten-fifteen in the evening. And thus to court.

A whole week of plaintiff testimony — odors, stinks, smells, awful sickening, horrible, horrendous, insomnia, asthma, vomiting, devalued property, lost sales, blighted community. I was convinced.

Then came the defense. By this time the judge was a bit irritated. He had hoped to handle the entire trial in two days. A whole week for the plaintiff. He complained:

"This trial is taking too long. There are other cases pending." Then with knifing sweetness the defense, through its lawyer, spoke, "I would remind the court that the previous week has been utilized by the plaintiff. I hope the defense may not be allowed any shorter time than that allotted the plaintiff."

The judge knows all that, but doesn't like it any better. And then the defense, benevolently, "In order to cooperate with the court may I state I have only one witness at this time and one hour may be sufficient for his examination."

"Bombshell." The prosecuting attorney is all alert. The judge throws off his lethargy. The air crackles with "Look Out."

The defense: "I call Mr. Hodges, the plant superintendent."

After the usual preliminaries, the attorney asked the unruffled Mr. Hodges: "Were you at the plant during any portion of the day or night of September 2nd?

Answer: "No."

Question: "Or the 1st?"

Answer: "No."

Question: "Or any other day of the first week of September or any day of the following week?"

Answer: "No."

Question: "Are you able to state from your employee records if any other persons were present during that period?"

Answer: "Only one day and one night watchman."

Question: "From your production records can you inform the court if there was a single pound of unworked material on the premises during that period?"

Answer: "There was no flesh left unworked."

Question: "Now, Mr. Hodges, will you tell the court why you and none of your workers were on duty from September the 1st to the 17th; why no work materials were on hand, and why there could not possibly have been any odors?"

Answer: "That is the period that we were completely closed down for all worker vacations."

The defense rested.

The case was dismissed, as it should have been.

But, but, you want to know, "How about the odors at the wedding?" "Were they not real?" Quite real. If you will refer to the journal of the sanitary department of that city for September 10th, you will find the answer in this entry:

> "The basin behind the Charles Street dam across Spencer Creek was drained on the 1st to permit the repair of a gas main traversing near the Charles Street bridge. Drying sludge banks led to offensive odors particularly during the night of the 2nd. Refilling of the basin began at noon on the 3rd."

So there you are!

Some sort of boon is claimed for restraint in escorting you about the fringes of the offensive trades. If by chance you have developed any fondness for them, go out and do your own olfactory investigations.

Chapter 16

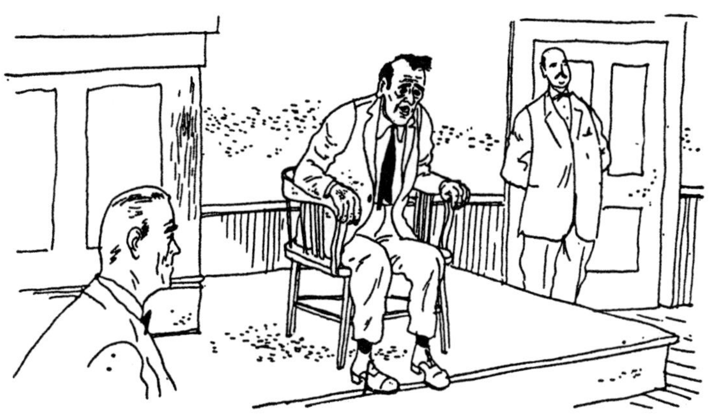

Chlorine and Chicanery

COMPARATIVELY few persons have been called upon to serve as a witness in any court trial. Many of the remainder speculate as to the "coaching" of witnesses by trial lawyers in getting ready for the trial. Some persons with a fine sense of honor would like to believe there exists between the prospective witness and the lawyer who proposes to use him, a complete aloofness. That is a gallant fantasy. Seldom does a witness take the chair without some interviewing. "Coaching" is scarcely the appropriate term in straightforward trial preparations.

These conferences are more for the education of the lawyer than of the witness. The witness may answer only what he may be asked, so that the lawyer must determine the trend of his inquiries. He is more concerned in the language best suited to emphasize or de-emphasize facts.

Language is much more important in a jury trial than in a trial before a judge. In an assumed trial for lead poisoning the plaintiff witnesses will be asked to stress "poisoning" over and over, since "poisoning" jars the jury; but the defense will resort to "plumbism," a term meaning just the same but likely to roll off the jury with fewer implications of disaster. In an "odor" trial, the plaintiff will bear down on "stinks," while the defense will seek more gently to ride along on "scents."

This confession centers about my unpraiseworthy readying for testimony in one reasty court procedure. Well aware that my scorn still might have repercussions, the circumstances are decidely disguised.

The telephone rang in my office. The call was long distance from a city six hundred miles away. An attorney, Mr. Rheinstron, related that he represented a group of five patients with chlorine poisoning from a paper pulp plant and needed medical guidance. Would I aid him in the preparation for the first trial? I would.

Two days later I presented myself at Mr. Rheinstron's office. He was busy for the time being, but sent out to me the record folder and had me placed in a comfortable office to review this material. The wait was a fairly long one, so that I had sufficient time to scan the collection of legal and medical papers.

When finally I was invited into Mr. Rheinstron's office, I was greeted with apologies by a plump little man who at once took a cigar out of a box for himself, but did not offer me one. That was a bad start.

He launched into the plans for the coming trial.

"Four of my five chlorine poisoning cases are textbook cases. The fifth one is a little shaky, and by bad luck, the worst case is set for the first trial. That's why I need you. I pretty near could win the other four without any medical testimony, but if I lose this first one I might lose all in spite of their being open and shut cases. You, doctor, have been over the record of this case that starts tomorrow. What do you think of it?"

Already a little wary, I began to make plans to ease out of a situation that didn't ring quite true. I stated, "Mr. Rheinstron, I have gone over the record you sent out to me and there does not seem to be any suggestion of chronic chlorine poisoning in it. I fear I will not be able to go on the stand and make any statement in this claimant's behalf. I never take cases unless I'm well convinced that they have some merit. With your permission, I'll drop out of this case, and pay my own expenses to and from your city. You get somebody else."

With a feeling of great honorableness, I prepared to leave. The shrewd lawyer did not give up. He was hurt and resentful, which feelings he unsuccessfully tried to hide. With a show of mollifying me, he said,

"Doctor, possibly you're right in this case, but I've got to use this first case to build up a setting for the remaining four and better cases. Would you be willing, Doctor, to present to the court a general picture of industrial chlorine poisoning and the circumstances under which it might arise, without any reference to this claimant?"

This appeared reasonable.

Thus I walked into a trap. I was younger then. Every industrial hygienist worthy of that title must make that blunder a few times before he becomes legalistically cautelous. I learned from Mr. Rheinstron. Without my saying a word he made me appear to be aligned with a cause that I had unequivocally condemned.

Soon the trial began. Other physicians, possibly better informed, or at least less scrupulous than I, recited from the witness chair a variety of signs and symptoms of a disease, all of which were laid at the door of chlorine.

The plaintiff, who, had he believed his own medical witnesses, should have been making hasty arrangements for departure from this earthly sphere, was far from in extremis on the witness stand in describing his work duties and his dangerous exposures. Let him tell his own story:

"I worked before I got this disease with four or five other fellahs in the basement below the heater room. I pulled pulp. Over us was the beater vats where shredded paper was mixed up with water and some chemical that gives off chlorine. This chlorine takes all the color out of the scrap paper. They don't have no chlorine to speak of up there because there are suckers that take off the gas. After the beating is done and the color is white, the water is drawn off. The stock is then dumped down to us. We don't make paper, we just make stock to ship to more paper plants. I pulled the stock, drippin' wet out of the chutes onto the floor. The other fellahs worked out more water and then pile it up."

"The gas," continued the afflicted one, after a drink of water, "was bad. Always bad, but sometimes worser. You couldn't see it but you could smell it. It was worse in the chutes than in the room, but plenty there too. It was chlorine gas."

Here somebody objected and wanted to know how he knew it was "chlorine." The witness fumbled around, mostly claiming that everybody knew it was chlorine. Mr. Rheinstron obligingly came to the rescue and shouted, "It will be established by other witnesses that it was chlorine all right."

Then back to the main recital:

"When I first went there it just made me cough and burnt my eyes. Somebody told me I'd get used to it. I tried to get used to it and for a while I thought I was. It was when the big slugs came through that it got me. Had to run plumb outside to get my breath. After about two years, I coughed all the time. Coughed all night every night. My chest hurt. Then I got asthma. Couldn't lie in bed. Had to sit on a chair half my night. Had six or eight doctors. They didn't do me any good. Bought medicine at the drug store—anything anybody told me was good. Some helped, some made me worser. After a while they took me to a hospital and made pictures of my lungs. Now they tell me I got the 'TB's.' All I know I haven't been to work for more than a year. Spent every dollar I had."

That's the kind of story that wins the jury. Mr. Rheinstron was smugly happy. I suspect that witness had been coached—but he forgot to cough. An oversight.

At a recess, I stated to Mr. Rheinstron, "I will be in much better position to describe this industrial operation if I might see the defendant's plant with my own eyes. Maybe this is a dangerous trade." I was beginning to like my trap.

The attorney replied, "As soon as we resume I will ask for a court order authorizing us to visit the plant."

The request was made and resistance quickly appeared. The court refused the request on the grounds that it would lead to the invasion of private rights and property. Privately Mr. Rheinstron said,

"Don't be disturbed. We will ask again tomorrow. Sooner or later the defense will want some favor. Then they'll be willing to trade."

Two more days passed. Step by step the jury was led to believe that a great injury had been done a neglected workman, that his health had been impaired, that his ability to support his family had been lost, no cure, totally and permanently disabled. During the fourth morning, I was not in the courtroom, having gone to a medical library, searching for additional toxicological materials.

A telephone call came to the library. Mr. Rheinstron was elated.

"Finally," he said, "the defense has granted us permission to inspect their plant. The court has adjourned for the afternoon for this purpose. We are to leave almost immediately. Come right over to the office. This plant is eighty-nine miles away."

Pleased with this prospect, I rushed to the attorney's office, expressing some dignified equivalent of "Let's go, let's go."

But the attorney was in no great hurry. A little leisurely he interviewed several waiting clients, then, with a temporary show of hurry and apology for the delay, we started. By this time it was one o'clock in the afternoon. Soon the attorney was reminded by his appetite that he had had no breakfast and no lunch and that he just could not make the trip without some food. I suggested a hurried sandwich or two to be eaten in the car. This plan did not suit the attorney. We ate well cooked steaks and fried potatoes, which consumed one of our precious hours. I expressed the desire to see this plant if possible during daylight and while operating. The procrastinating

Mr. Rheinstron thought the plant operated on three shifts and that we would have no difficulty. By three o'clock, we had covered only forty miles when Mr. Rheinstron suddenly decided that an engineer, later to be called as a witness, by all means also should inspect the offending factory. We retraced thirty miles of our journey. All this delay was beyond my understanding. The engineer was located working in his garden. He had to change his clothes. Another half hour was lost. Purporting to make up for lost time, Mr. Rheinstron, the driver, attempted a "short cut." It might be guessed that on this short cut the car broke down. By this time, resigned to any happening, I gave up the fight.

Not until nine o'clock did we reach the plant. No night shift was working. Mr. Rheinstron pointed out that all arrangements had been made by the defendant attorneys and that we would be expected, even at this late hour. He asked the engineer and myself to wait in the car while he hunted up the "night superintendent."

Soon he returned with the night watchman, with a lantern. All the lights of the plant were then turned on. An adequate opportunity was provided to see the machinery, the storage of treated pulp — every process, the furnace equipment.

At the end of an hour, my observations were completed, the notes made sufficient. As a last step, we were walking, I with the night watchman, to a sludge pile on the outside of the factory building where unusable stock was piled in small windrows. During this trip, the night watchman inquired, "Where is it you're going to build your factory?" This seemed irrelevant. Maybe the night watchman was confusing me with some other member of the group. He repeated, "Where is it that you're going to build this new factory of yours?"

I replied, "I beg your pardon, possibly I did not understand you. I'm not going to build any factory. I'm a doctor. I'm a witness in the trial involving this plant. It was arranged for me to inspect it."

The now frightened night watchman put down his lantern and turned on Mr. Rheinstron saying, "Didn't you give me ten dollars,

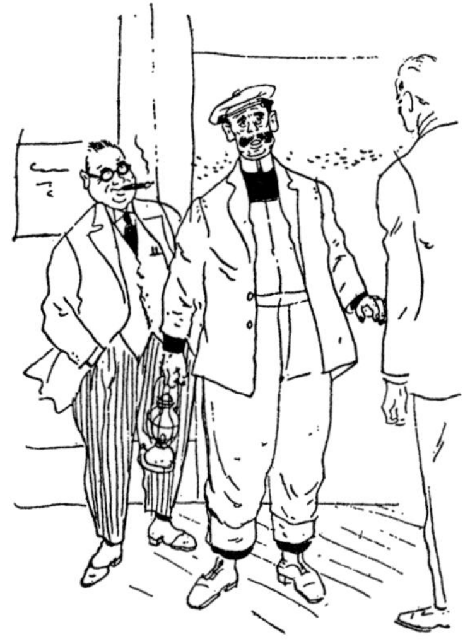

telling me that this man was going to build a paper plant somewhere out West? Now he's telling me that he doesn't know anything about any new factory and that he is a part of this trial going on upstate. I'll lose my job."

Mr. Rheinstron was undisturbed. "Don't be upset by anything I told you. We'll get out now." We did.

Back in the car, Mr. Rheinstron was delighted with himself. I was furious. The full details of the plan were now becoming quite apparent.

The court in truth had adjourned for half a day, not for the purpose named, but to permit the judge to attend a funeral. No permission had been given by the defendants for any examination of their plant. There never had been any intention of arriving at the plant while it was in operation, and all of the delays were planned and scheduled. Even the accident had been prefabricated. A wire had been attached to some portion of the motor with the other end tied in under the instrument panel. It was only necessary for Mr. Rheinstron to pull on this wire to cause a breakdown. It was all nicely planned and executed.

Mr. Rheinstron, still pleased with himself, stated that no court ever questioned the method through which evidence was obtained.

"Now," he said, "we are really in position to lick them. We have seen every portion of the plant."

"You won't lick them with this witness," I replied indignantly. "If called on the stand, I will fully state just what has taken place tonight and show my unwillingness to participate in any such affairs. I'm through."

Here then is one way that evidence is obtained. That it is unusual and disgusting is granted.

Oh yes! The trial jury awarded this claimant fifteen thousand dollars.

Today this litigant is a truck driver for a coal company; the physical examination card, stored in the coal company's office, has a ring around that symbol which means "Physically fit for any job." Mr. Rheinstron knows this. He explains, "You remember I told you he wasn't one of my good claims from that plant."

Somewhere over the years I learned there were no other four claimants from that plant. I learned about lawyers from Mr. Rheinstron.

Chapter 17

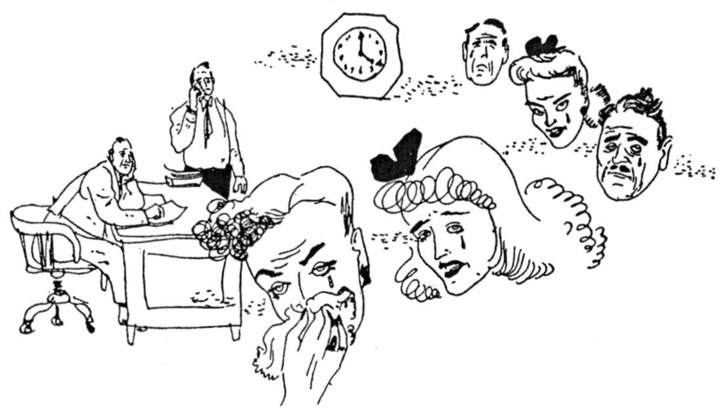

The Four O'Clock Mystery

Every physician is a detective. The cause of a disease is the criminal. The diagnosis but names the criminal. The "arrest" may be far ahead.

So, into my medical detective headquarters, came the assistant superintendent of the Kelsey Bookbinding Co. seeking detective services. After introductions, he pictured the crime, beginning with an apology.

"Maybe what I am about to tell you is foolish and you may think that we are a lot of lunkheads out at the plant, but we do seem to be in trouble and we can't make heads nor tails out of what seems to be going on. At any rate, Doctor, let me tell you what is happening and maybe you can help us.

"Every afternoon during the hot weather at about five minutes past four, all of our office force on the first floor of the north wing of our building are suddenly irritated about the eyes, nose and throat until they are in a complete stew. Their eyes are genuinely inflamed and even the next morning some few eyes are still red and apparently sore. There are usually twenty-seven girls in this section of the work and four men, all working under a supervisor with an office in the same area.

"At first we pooh-poohed these complaints and attributed all this jumpiness to tiredness from hard work during the summer season. Especially it seemed ridiculous that any disturbance should come at exactly the same time of day three or four minutes after four o'clock. Then we stationed two of our very dependable and mature men from another floor in this first floor section and sure enough on the minute these men, who are quite unlikely to be taken in by any hysterical mania, were gassed or poisoned, or at least something happened to them which made them very uncomfortable."

Mr. Kelsey paused to appraise my degree of credulity.

"For the next two or three days we looked around to see if by chance any railroad train passed by at four o'clock. We are close to a main line on one side of our building. We thought that the gases in the smoke from a locomotive might be responsible. No locomotive has been in sight during the past two days at four o'clock. Someone then suggested that traffic on the Boulevard might markedly increase at four o'clock, and that this condition might be due to increased quantities of motor gases. We put two men on the job of clocking automobiles and trucks, one each being responsible for travel in the two directions, but we found, at least during the past two days, that traffic is considerably less at four o'clock than at four-thirty and much less at four than at five o'clock. Now we have no explanation and we have come to you. We have no medical department of our own, being a small-sized organization. We don't even have a nurse. Would you care to come out and see if you can help us?"

The next day I spent from one o'clock until three-thirty in the afternoon in the department described by the assistant superintendent, interviewing various workers. The portion of the plant involved was not given over to bookbinding, but instead to the usual office work of the company, bookkeepers, stenographers, secretaries, the cashier's office, and similar office activities. There were noted a few adding machines, dictaphones, a small photostatic outfit, but no operation that might be the source of any outstanding irritant.

All of the workers consulted gave substantially the same story. Every afternoon since the hot spell had begun, and shortly after four o'clock and at no other time during the day, their eyes began to burn, tears to flow. At the same time, the nasal passages were similarly affected, some complained of sneezing and coughing, one or two of nosebleed, a greater number of nausea. During the past two or three weeks, a few women had fainted. Two had quit work. Knowing that the irritant would arrive in the air shortly after four o'clock, the present practice was to leave this work area about fifteen or twenty minutes, going to other portions of the building—restrooms, washrooms, etc. That afternoon all workers agreed to stay at their work points in order that I might have full opportunity to make observations.

At four o'clock, various whistles from neighboring factories blew, marking the end of the factory workers' day. At that moment, the air in the workroom under investigation in no-wise suggested any extraneous content.

At four minutes after four, one girl exclaimed: "There it is!"

A few seconds later, I was aware of a definite irritant. My own eyes watered and burned. I sneezed freely. My throat seemed dry and seared. Several girls moved to open windows. A major number, with handkerchiefs over their noses and mouths, abandoned the room. I didn't blame them. The disturbance was real. In a few minutes, the irritant disappeared, but as I went about the room all eyes were inflamed slightly, eyelids swollen and red. They recognized in me a champion and were delighted that at least their complaints were being heeded.

The next morning I checked over every portion of the plant's operations. Nothing in the normal course of work possibly could have accounted for this four o'clock onslaught. A portion of the morning was spent in the basement, which, in fact under the north wing, was not a full basement, but a half-cellar given over to a tangle of pipelines, tanks and wires.

Even at this time in this cellar area an irritant gas was present, the nature of which I suspected, but I waited until four o'clock. As much on schedule as an eclipse, the irritant appeared. In this sub-cellar, the gas was almost overpowering, asphyxiating. I left as rapidly as possible. I, at least, knew the entryway if not the origin of the difficulty.

Inquiry was made as to the absence of a full basement under this portion of the building. Promptly the reply came, "There's an old-time sewer, long abandoned by the city, running under that portion of the building and so near the surface that we couldn't build a basement."

We found various openings into this old sewer, broken pipes, a manhole, and apparently one or two small caved-in sections. The answer was becoming apparent. Undoubtedly the offending gas was hydrogen sulfide. Most persons believe that this stinking gas always warns of its presence by its odor. Paradoxically the more this gas is present, less of the odor is noticed. When it may be smelled, ordinarily it will not irritate. Half the problem was solved, but why was the difficulty limited to four o'clock?

At the City Engineer's office, I sought out blueprints of this old sewer. The engineering assistant was careful to emphasize that this sewer had been abandoned—that no permits were issued for any connections to it. But, I inquired, "Do any factories anywhere along its extent still use it for sewage discharge?"

Reluctantly the engineer replied, "Undoubtedly some of the very old plants still are hooked up with this sewer. We no longer have any record."

Armed with the blueprint, and with the knowledge that this sewer had been condemned in 1913, I began to trace out its course. Most of the buildings along its course clearly had been built since 1913. Here and there might be observed cornerstones or, above door markings, 1922, 1917, 1926, but half a mile away from the book-

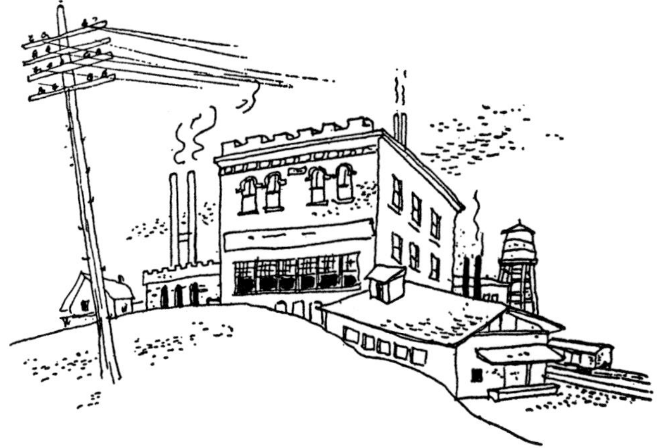

bindery was a large and ancient tannery. Here was the probable disturber of peace and comfort in the bookbindery.

In the tannery, I inquired for the plant engineer, who was most cooperative, and of him I asked this question,

"Just before your plant force quits work, what is done that is not done at any other hour of the day?"

After a little, he made reply.

"We open up the cocks on all of the tanning vats out of which hides have been pulled that day. Altogether, we have several dozen tanning vats containing hides in various stages of tanning, but the schedule is such that every day that we operate we are able to empty from four to six vats. When empty of hides, the tanning liquor is no longer valuable, and this we turn into the sewer every afternoon just before quitting time. This is the job of one of the straw bosses."

Mystery no more. Tanning liquors contain enough decomposing organic materials, from hides and skins, to generate dangerous quantities of hydrogen sulfide. The hotter the weather, the more freely this gas leaves the water in which it is dissolved.

"Simple," you complain just a little disappointed.

"Quite so," I admit freely, still a little pleased with myself. "Nothing is really hard after you get to it. The solutions by better detectives of famous murders and kidnappings become equally simple after they are spread as headlines across the newspaper."

Always when I relate this minor event in a lecture room or auditorium, someone pipes up, "What did you do after that to get rid of the gas?"

That was simple, too. Tannery officials, a little frightened maybe, graciously agreed to discharge no waste until five o'clock rather than three-thirty. A few days later the bookbindery arranged to seal off all openings into the sewer. After that, no more teary eyes at four o'clock — no more gas, no more mystery.

Indeed simple!

Chapter 18

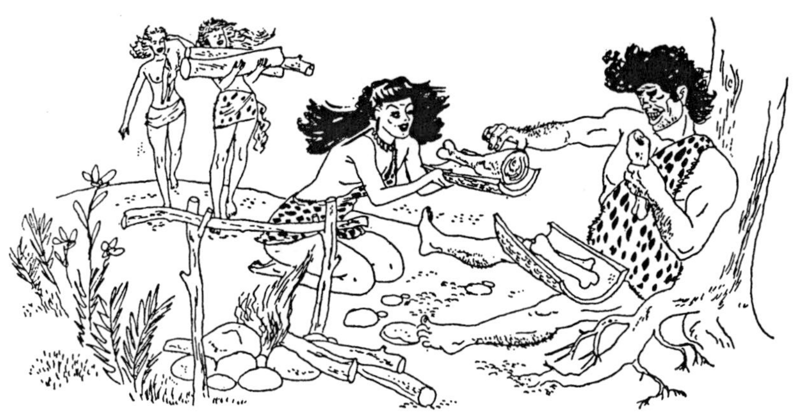

Women at Work

EVERY generation has to make a few discoveries all for itself. One of these discoveries is that women work. In that remarkable book of Ramazzini's, nearly two hundred and fifty years old, now worthy of ungrudging tribute, many references are made to "wenches" at work. In the days of Ramazzini's early translators, "wench" was a polite word implying a little more adulthood than our currently used "moppet." Nowadays "wench" has ignominiously sunk to the level of "strumpet." So hastily, and with apologies if already offense has been given, I ease away from the designation of the old master and embrace "women."

So early as 1921, I discovered the valorous services of women in industry as a continuous contribution, and not merely linked with the industrial upsurges of war and other commotions. In that year with Dorothy Minster, an associate, a study was made of pregnant working women.

Women have always worked. The truth is that women worked

before man, tamed him, taught him how to work, and put him to work. Man became so successful at work that clever woman eased out from many of her former tasks and let man have them.

Although millions of women for decades have engaged in work other than about their own households, many masculine die-hards are fully convinced that they have no place in industry. Possibly this stems from the legendary Paul Bunyan, wherein these mysterious beings called "women" are charged with wrecking the logging industry — at least Paul Bunyan's kind of timbering. Gallantly denying such havoc-working in all industry, it may not be claimed that women at work do not make special problems, production problems, labor problems, medical problems, group problems, individual problems — as in the case of Beatrice — Beatrice, the bucker.

A bucker, in case you are uncertain, holds a brick shaped bat of metal against the reverse side of sheet metal being riveted by her partner on the obverse side. Beatrice was a woman of average height — that means she was four and a half inches shorter than her ample counterpart. More importantly it means that, in the application of her bucking iron, elbows and forearms rested more heavily about her right breast. Beatrice developed cancer in this right breast, which in itself is not remarkable since some tens of thousands of women have developed breast tumors without influence of any work. It may be doubted that trauma of this character frequently plays a significant part in cancer production; but the number of compensation claims that arise is impressive.

In Beatrice's case there was no contention on her part that cancer had been caused by work. The difficulty was the light hearted and complete denial that a cancer existed or possibly could exist. In the presence of frank carcinoma, attested by the best of surgeons, Beatrice sweetly but with great finality pointed out that she could never have cancer.

"Quite impossible," she said.

In a surge of astrological language which I am sure I am mixing, there was so much of it, she poured out,

"I am under Aries with Cancer rising and in the house of Cancer I am protected by Jupiter. This means I can't have cancer, at least not now."

"You doctors," she continued, "mean well. But just forget me. You don't understand the unseen powers that protect me."

This represents no condemnation of those persons who elect to place some store by astrology, but Beatrice's language lost some of its eloquence when she gesticulated with her left hand while holding in her right hand a tragically cancerous breast. We, her doctors, better trusting our own eyesight and fingers than the influence of planets in their courses, could not agreeably fall in line with her plan. Away she went, possibly for further advices and treatment by the astrologer.

Beatrice died of neglected carcinoma of the breast. If unfortunately she may make no further difficulty, millions of other women workers will provide a greater share of health problems than any equivalent number of men. Women, always mysterious (mystery being their chief tool of power) carry this quality to work benches and machines, all to the end that fabulous stories have grown up around them.

One of the fantastic beliefs, but not widely accepted, is that the touch of women's hands on metal during their menstrual period leads to rusting. The truth is the touch of sweaty fingers of either men or women at all times will stain or mildly corrode some metals. The claim against the flowing woman would have you believe that in some magical fashion the acidity of the perspiration is altered in this state, that the quantity of salt as a constituent is modified so that literally the biblical terminology of "unclean" takes on industrial significance. In behalf of women functioning as nature intended, let it be written that there is no shred of proof in the charge against them. Does every woman's finger-touch stain highly polished metal? Yes, indeed, but so does the touch of every man.

There perhaps remain a few work places where the very presence, even on a momentary basis, of a woman bodes ill. In mining operations in particular long has prevailed the belief that for every woman who enters the mine a death will occur among the miners. If by chance some woman enters any one of many mines this fact is bruited about rapidly, and the miners leave their diggings for the day, hoping thereby to break the spell of evil influence. While it is not necessary to leave this country to see this superstition in operation, you possibly may see it at its best or worst among the Indian silver miners at Taxco in Mexico.

Understandably enough, there is a filament of actuality in the dangers of a pretty woman visiting a factory when her presence is unusual. For the time being the usual safety precautions are tossed aside and the most foolish happenings arise. Once I conducted a young lady through a metals trade plant, explaining various operations and describing different types of machines. At one machine I pointed out an unguarded set of gears, obviously dangerous, and innocently observed that if by chance the worker nearby carelessly moved his hand two feet away from his usual point of operation, disaster might take place. Proving my point and following some utterly unexplainable suggestion, the worker did just that, with the loss of several fingers.

Factories for the most part were built for men, not for women. The level of work benches is too high, tool handles are too large, reaching distances to machine parts are too great for women. They were all built for men. The height of a kitchen sink was decided by woman's anatomical requirements. But when she replaces men in industry nearly always there is a need for scaling down of work arrangements. A four-inch standing platform provided for women workers on occasion may save the job against the claim of accidents among women, undue fatigue, frequent absenteeism, and such.

Men have found it difficult to accept women workers as equals chiefly because women themselves for decades have fostered the belief that they were peculiarly different from men, delicate creatures unusually susceptible to many kinds of diseases, including some occupational diseases. They persuaded legislatures to make laws for their especial protection, and the Supreme Court of the United States has handed down learned opinions insisting upon the fragility of women workers.

Without cavil, and quickly before I am attacked as a disbeliever, I place in the record the recognition that on a physical basis there are a few definite feminine handicaps. These are not merely on a pound for pound basis. Differences in sport capacities are illuminating. The best woman's baseball team is not the equal of the best man's nine — but nobody suggests that the women outfielders be supplied chairs.

Many of the special provisions for women workers are unnecessary, often foolish, and more often serve as a deterrent to woman's progress toward industrial equality with men.

One group of all-knowing club women inspecting a candy factory, and squealing with delight at the end over the luscious confections furnished with only the remote thought of currying favor, had discovered one group of girls working in the cold room chocolate-coating chilled centers destined to become liquid centers for the consumer. These girls were warmly and comfortably maintained. In the heat of summer their work was an envied boon. Imagine the difficulty of coating a spoonful of liquid center. No less the helpful ladies earnestly urged that the refrigeration room be heated. Everyone accepted this wisdom with straight faces until the ladies safely were on their way — then factory-wide laughter.

Without truckling to the ladies, but without carrying the matter too far, there are many reasons for tagging the female as physically superior to man. Man is the weaker of the sexes. Without comparison, the farmer may be quoted when in pride over his team of horses, he expresses preference in saying, "The grey mare is the better horse." Woman's physical forte is stamina. Under many circumstances where men and women are equally exposed to direful conditions, woman is the last survivor. This may be accepted at law. In the case of man and wife dying in a fire without there being any prospect of determining the order of death, some courts, in their desire equitably to dispose of property, will assume that the man dies first. Of a group of men and women exposed in a boat, who survives? The women or a woman — not always of course, but often enough to attract attention. But, you say, the men chivalrously gave their coats to the ladies, nor did they exhaust themselves with rowing. Maybe so, but let the boat capsize, who reaches shore if anybody? Plenty of times — the ladies. And yet some of us in derision refer to the "weaker sex."

One of the amazing features of women as industrial workers is their dirtiness. It is hard to believe that three times as much janitor work is necessitated in some work places for women as for men. Unfortunately this may not be attributed to a demand for three times the cleanliness that men demand. Baldly stated, the reverse is true, Women, the very symbol of cleanliness of the home, little carry this quality into work places. If there be doubt, let the doubter visit the respective washrooms of men and women performing the same duties.

One of the engaging terms that have grown up around woman's work in industry is "race poisoning." Obviously a race poison is one that may involve offspring. For women in industry it is conceded that there are numerous substances that so harm the mother before or during pregnancy that there may arise spontaneous abortion, stillbirth or a defective output.

Lead is regarded as a race poison since undeniably harm may be done to the unborn child. Benzene falls into the same category since damaging hemorrhage from women's generative organs may interfere with the normal events of pregnancy. Radium finds a place in this same grouping, since it appears to be true that the ravages of radium on the mother illy may serve the interests of children.

Of course, there are race poisons, and we should never countenance a work world in which work conditions interfere with the well-being of the unborn or lately born. But women workers may not preempt this term. It is not a sex-linked affair. The children of women who have never worked may be the victims of race poison through damage to the working father. Again pointing to our always handy example of lead poisoning, it may be proved that the germ cell damage in the father fully may equal any corresponding damage to the mother, but since the mother plays a so much greater part in the child-production function, the onus, if there be onus, unequitably becomes her lot.

The answer from the practical industrial hygienist's point of view always is that neither for women nor men should there be tolerated work conditions harmful to themselves or to any offspring, and whatever work conditions, with few exceptions, are desirable for women workers are equally desirable for men. There is scant justification for any separate standards for women workers. If you must have an example of the exception, find it in the difference in number of toilet seats respectively required for men and women and the reason therefor.

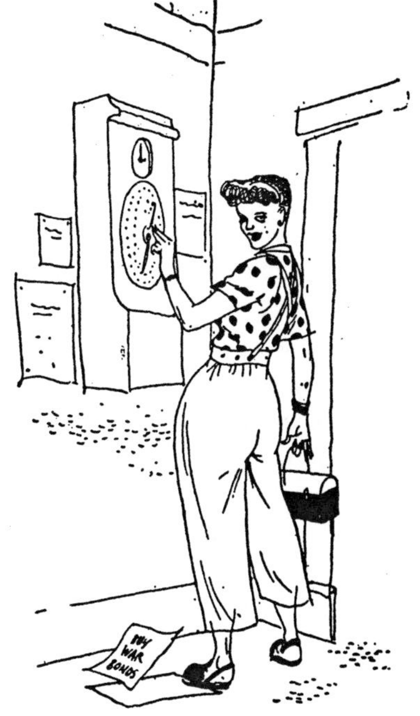

While we are eying women workers, albeit without comprehensiveness, it may be well to have a look at that troublesome matter, the double absentee frequency of women over men. On any average day some eight per cent of women may be missing from their desks, work benches and machines, but only four per cent of men, and this on a basis of a forty-hour work week. Should the work week be increased to forty-four a mounting absenteeism may be expected. Why this difference?

Learned ones may present statistical arrangements proving to their satisfaction, if not to mine, that women are doubly susceptible to respiratory infections, more susceptible to occupational diseases, or hampered by the menstrual function. All this is challenged.

The chief reason for woman's increased absenteeism, unkindly put, is related to the requirements of household duties, her deeper interest in her household, her delight in deliberate shopping, her willingness to spend unconscionable hours at the beauty parlor.

There are still other reasons. Woman's clothing actually may promote a higher incidence of respiratory diseases, not that this represents a fundamental susceptibility difference. The same applies to dietary habits. But of greater importance is the attitude of the employer or supervisor. Having been educated through some decades that women are the delicate members of the work force, they are shooed away to their homes with the first sneeze or sniffle, while men are merely given a dirty look and the casual hope that maybe tomorrow they will be well again.

This book claims no right to draw morals or conclusions, but in this damning situation in which women are saddled with double the load of the high costs of absenteeism, it is possible to point out that much of it is artificial and not any result of fundamental physiological shortcomings of the ladies.

The structure of woman's body never was designed for weight-lifting. Moreover, no modest woman, wearing woman's kind of clothes, can with mental comfort for herself and without the hilarity of nearby males ever assume the best physiologic position for weight-lifting. This is just one reason for the advocacy of slacks. In the midst of a lot of the pro and con about the inevitability of some weight-lifting for most women in industry there came the real answer to the weight-lifting problem both for men and women. Industry has found it economic and expedient to introduce, wherever required, small cunning weight-lifting devices, simple in operation and a changer of women's status in industry. With these devices on hand it now becomes possible to maintain that seventy and perhaps even eighty per cent of all industry's tasks may be performed by women, sometimes better than, but more often as well as men. No less, women may perform the tasks.

With a lot of admiration for the capacities of women who enter industry and replace men on an almost equal footing, the temptation is to go on and on in an effort to break down the traditional objection to women as workers. This seems to be unnecessary. There is no likelihood that women will replace men as workers in industry in dominating numbers when the need is no longer acute. Woman's heart is not in industry, however loyal she may be to its temporary needs. She is likely to step aside, except for that large group of women who are self-supporters or breadwinners for families. However, there is no possibility that we may revert to that state reflected by the revealing Biblical language descriptive of the virtuous woman, which includes these words: "Her husband is known in the gates, where he sitteth among the elders of the land" (sounds like he was going in for politics); "she maketh fine linen, selleth it and delivereth girdles unto the merchants." It is unfortunate that, at the day and time of this writing, she cannot get even one girdle for herself.

Chapter 19

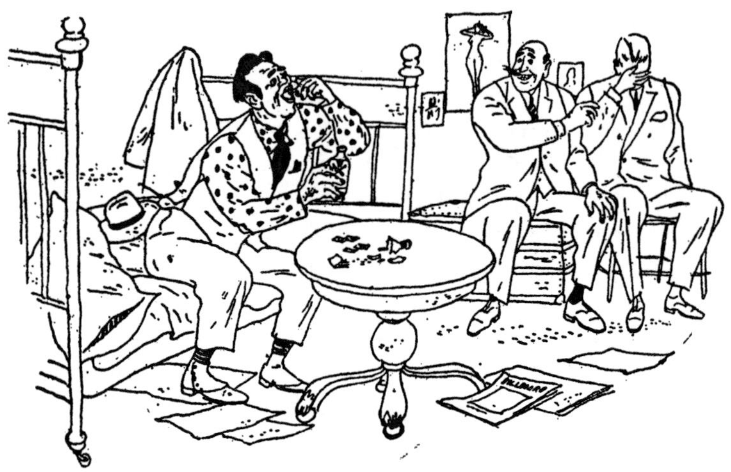

The Man Who Refused to be Poisoned

IN COURTROOMS I have suffered many defeats. The worst routing in a courtroom was at the hands, or more rightly the stomach, of a moronic witness, brought in by an obstreperous employer who was contesting the valid claim of one of his employees for formaldehyde poisoning. This employer was an undertaker, and the claimant had been an assistant who aided in embalming, using formalin, which is a watery solution of formaldehyde gas.

This assistant had been damaged by breathing the formaldehyde gas from the formalin solution, repeatedly used in a small cubbyhole of an embalming room without any ventilation. In my testimony I had described his various symptoms and the findings made by me on examination. With scientific propriety, I had emphasized the presence of several small lung abscesses, which disturbance is common in cases of severe chronic poisoning by inhalation.

While most of the legal procedure dealt with the effect of formaldehyde gases on the body, I was led into a series of questions about the poisonous properties of liquid formalin by mouth. I stated that a tablespoonful might kill a person, and that no person is known to have recovered after drinking more than two ounces of the full strength material. This type of formalin injury does not occur in industry, since men and women in industry working with formalin do not go about drinking it. However, formalin deaths are well known to coroners' pathologists following accidental intake and suicide.

The lethal dose cited by me was amply substantiated by many publications on toxicology.

On cross examination the employer's attorney asked of me,

"What would you expect if here in this courtroom I produced a man who in our presence would drink half a pint of full strength formalin?"

With uncautious certainty, I predicted that he would be affected in a few minutes and unfailingly be dead within a few hours.

Soon, just such a witness was put on the stand. There was produced a half-pint bottle of formalin, manufactured by a reputable pharmaceutical house with the seal unbroken. The witness was a stocky, stolid foreigner, little concerned in what to some of us was a dramatic and criminal procedure. The lawyer said, "This man will now drink the full contents of this bottle and you'll see that it does him no harm."

After the seal was broken, I was asked to agree that it was formalin, which I did, although I could not agree to any strength of solution and had no knowledge as to other constituents of the bottle's contents. I protested the wickedness of allowing any person to risk his life through this proposed nefarious act. The court did not object, and the witness without ostentation drank the entire lot of this deadly poison. I withdrew as far as possible in the courtroom to make clear that I was no abetting party. Confidently I expected this man to collapse. He did nothing of the sort. With a little showmanship, he smacked his lips with the last drop and said, "I'll drink another bottle if anybody wants me to."

He didn't die. Nothing happened. No antidote was administered.

The elated lawyer turned to the court and said, "It must be quite clear that formalin is not poisonous. By the statements of the medical expert in this room about the high degree of toxicity of formalin, this man, if any of those statements were true, would now be writhing in agony or unconscious, and yet anyone can see that he is quite unharmed. He has volunteered to drink more should we request it, thus proving that formalin is as harmless as drinking water."

All this required a considerable period of time and, from all experience, this witness should have been in agony. I was dumbfounded. The judge looked at me as though concealing shame over a physician who would trump up a lot of lying evidence in behalf of a malingerer who had never been sick from formaldehyde action and could not possibly have been harmed by it. Had its harmlessness not been demonstrated before his very eyes? The case was lost.

The decision was not immediately reached, but the impression had been made. At a later time, a verdict unfavorable to my patient was rendered.

Then it was I hunted up the undertaker's lawyer and inquired,

"Where did you run across that formaldehyde drinker?"

Gleefully he replied, "I found him in the sideshow of a petty circus, but he lives here in this city. Day by day he goes around to various bars, wherever he can get a hearing, and he'll agree to drink a cup of formalin for a quarter. He does this every day. Nothing ever happens. I have his address. Would you like to go down and see him?"

I was anxious to do this, but I protested, "You know that formalin is a deadly poison."

"Yes," he agreed, "for most people, but I'm a lawyer. I'll do anything to win my case, and we certainly won over you. Your testimony wasn't worth a nickel after my man put on his show. He's got a lot of other tricks, too. Come on, let's go and see him."

At this man's sordid quarters, he agreed to eat razor blades, swallow needles, eat a handful of glass and drink a cupful of formalin for a dollar. I refused either to furnish the dollar or any of the dangerous materials, but the lawyer did.

Within my own eyesight and without a possibility of subterfuge, this freak chewed up and swallowed six used safety razor blades (thus solving his personal problem of how to dispose of used razor blades); swallowed unbroken, one by one, a package of cambric needles, all of the broken glass from one electric light bulb — and washed all this down with a highball of formalin.

I examined the interior of his mouth. The mucous membranes were abnormally white, thick, and leatherish. There were two or three tiny bloody spots from nicks of the glass or metal. Nothing more.

The freak asked that I hold a blazing match under his forearm. This I did for a full fifteen seconds, with the blaze directly in contact with the skin. He did not flinch and laughed at his superiority over ordinary man. His skin was not damaged, and later the next day when I examined him there were no blisters or signs of burn.

At this point, he asked me to cut his skin with a remaining razor blade, stating that he would demonstrate his ability to prevent bleeding. I refused thus to harm him, whereupon he slashed his own skin, making a cut about two inches in length and well into the skin if not through it. The injury was sufficient to produce profuse bleeding in the usual person. My miracle man snapped his fingers over the wound and commanded it not to bleed. Not a drop of blood appeared.

On the following day, armed with due legal releases and having been assured that daily he engaged in the body mutilations earlier demonstrated, I tolerated him to chew up and swallow metal behind a fluoroscope, in the presence of a few other physicians. Quite impersonally the faithful x-ray fluoroscope portrayed the passage of the metal into the stomach. X-ray films produced a permanent record of the event.

At a shortly later time, at the Academy of Medicine, after recounting my knowledge of this freak to the assembled members, assuring them that what I was about to do was but his daily practice, I permitted him to demonstrate his apparent utter non-response to acts that probably would have killed the usual person, and certainly would have been associated with profound damage. By a smug group of physicians assembled, I was roundly condemned for lending any degree of support to any mentally deficient person who might indulge in such destructive acts, despite my representation that these things constituted a daily performance and on occasion many times daily, and that I, in making a scientific presentation, was exhibiting nothing more than what might be expected to take place were this man on the stage. I was rebuked.

What is the explanation? I have none. Occasionally nature in her wisdom or folly bizarrely produces a creature whose tissues refuse to respond in the manner typical for normal persons. Scientifically this condition may be related to the well-known affection called syringomyelia — but that is a term and not an explanation. At any rate, this unfortunate, feeble-minded man, through his acts that represented his bid to fame, was utilized to defeat a meritorious court claim and to bring to me much chagrin.

Scientific curiosity, that impelling maid, goaded me into the desire to learn if truly he might be equally resistant to the highly deadly alkaloids such as strychnine. The freak was wholly willing, but his low mentality was his protection. No physician would take that step. A compromise was made on a lower level of toxicity. I wanted to determine if he might be entirely non-responsive to lead. Small quantities, such as barely might bring about minor lead colic in a normal person, would at most induce no great harm.

A deal was made whereby I was to put him in a hospital (this chiefly to prevent his daily show-off with formaldehyde) and pay him a small wage for his time. Insistently he made the demand that in addition I present him with the x-rays showing the razor blade metal in his stomach. This seemed fair enough and so I did — then and there. That was all he wanted. The lure of the circus got him. That night he disappeared.

Never another sight of him, but for years after, as this circus Aeneas went his way, I would receive occasional taunting news of a freak in a third-rate sideshow with a background of x-ray view boxes and, in them, my x-ray films.

Believe me, friend or foe, I really am not in the business of furnishing x-ray films for the ballyhoo of sideshows.

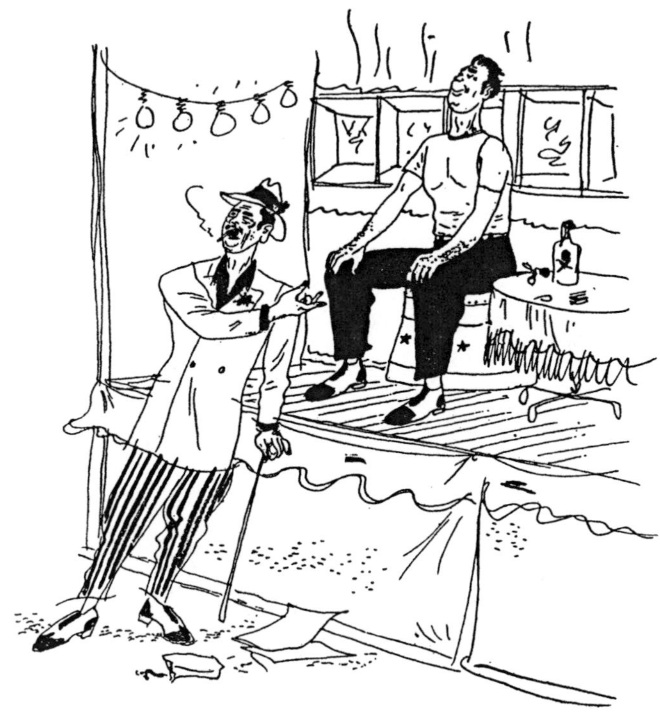

Chapter 20

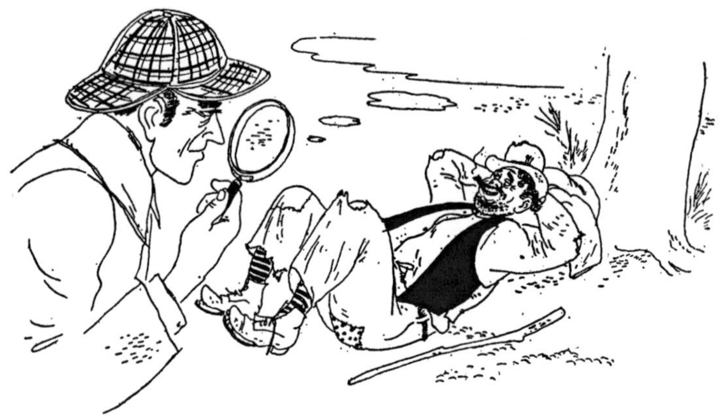

Medical Sideshow

HAVING just proclaimed my impeccability in connection with sideshows and their freaks, now to reveal my perversity, I am staging my own sideshow. A medical sideshow, but no freaks. Instead, some fifteen booths occupied by men and women workers who on their bodies have telltale markings of their jobs. These, by custom, are called work "stigmata," but that term harbors degrading implications — so, into the discard.

Any industrial physician with a flair for the dramatic, readily may gain a reputation for "second sight." A patient never before seen, walks in, partly unclad. Beyond salutation, not a word may be spoken until the doctor asks, "What sort of furnace work do you do?" or "How long were you a farmer?" or "When did you leave the Army?" His body or his speech or his garb may shout his trade. But, on with the show — "In this booth we have . . ."

The workman is examined when his legs are bare. The fronts of his thighs are criss-crossed with coarse red markings. There are none on the rear, few below the knees. Already this man has revealed his job. He is a furnace worker standing all day before some source of radiant heat. If the markings were prominent below the knee, and were it winter, that would be different. Then his checker-board skin pattern might derive from a stove or a fireplace at home. Without any questioning, the workman's trade is mentioned to him. He is puzzled. If you too are puzzled, thumb through any "skin book" until you find "dermatitis ab igne" — skin disease from fire.

On a streetcar opposite me is a workman. He is no acquaintance. I do not know where he is employed. We do not speak. I enter him in my mental little red book — "glass blower." "Why?" This workman told me with his teeth. In the midline his four incisors form a circle into which a button but not quite a dime might be inserted. Worn round by his blowpipe. He is an old timer. It takes years to gain this honorable badge of hard work. You may want to argue just a little and say, "Smoking his pipe did this." Not in this case. The wear of a pipe is apt to be oval, smaller, and more often on one side. Convinced?

At the movies, a few persons near me sniff the air, growl a little and move back four rows. I am not embarrassed lest I be the source of odors. I know the difficulty. The man next to me, a stranger, reeks of garlic — no, not garlic, but like garlic. I stay, for his crime is no greater than being a selenium worker. Selenium, tellurium, and rarely arsenic, betray those who work with them. The breath takes on more than a hint of garlic. In this case, I am willing to apply, "stigmata of work."

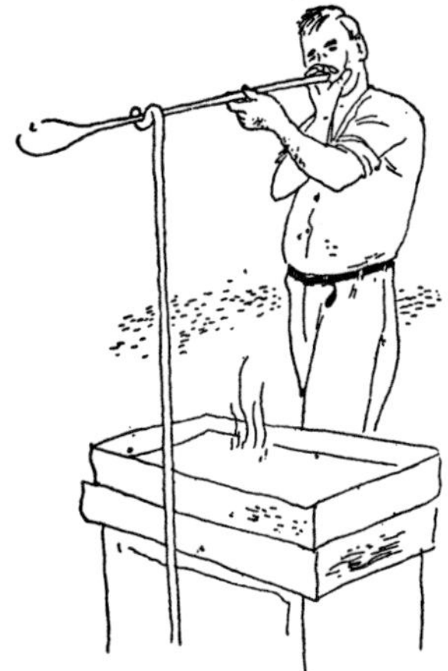

Waiting at my dentist's office, the victim in the chair is asked if I, a physician, may be permitted to see his teeth. He agrees. The dentist is trying to show me up. That's easy, but not this time. The patient discloses teeth well worn down evenly so. There is no decay. The gums are scarcely inflamed. There is no pain. "What," queries the dentist of me, "is this man's job?" "Acid worker," I suggest. "Right," says the dentist — a little disappointed.

It is time we garnered a few women for the sideshow. One woman holds her own record and knows that I have not examined it. She is a newcomer at the office. At once I inquire, "How long have you done aluminum polishing?" She looks first at me then at her attire. It is neat, clean street wear. No evidence there. But there is evidence. A few flecks of bright metal caught in her eyebrows reflect light. I pretend omnipotence, and she wonders if she is to believe it. Then the truth. Her mind is relieved and she adds, "You probably will find lots more on my scalp." There were, but none had anything to do with her trouble.

The erect, ruddy, young man said, "Good morning, sir. I think, sir, I may have a touch of the 'crabs.' Have had them before, sir." My reply was not irrelevant, "Did you have them in the Army?" He wasn't astonished. Neither are you.

An older woman, but still under forty, wanted an appointment. She entered, obviously dejected, and self rejected. Striking was her skin, wherever it might be seen. It was an even slaty blue — the whites of her eyes were blue. She was pathetic. A condition wholly beyond remedy. I knew the diagnosis, and she knew the diagnosis. As ever, I tried to put my best foot forward. "You have been a silver worker?" "No," she replied, "I am an inspector of fabrics, and have been for years." I was caught off balance. She saved me by adding, "I know what is going through your head, Doctor, but I got my silver given me for years by my own doctor for stomach

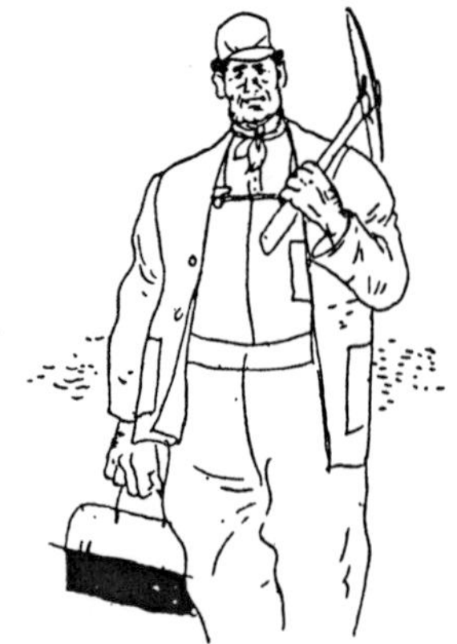

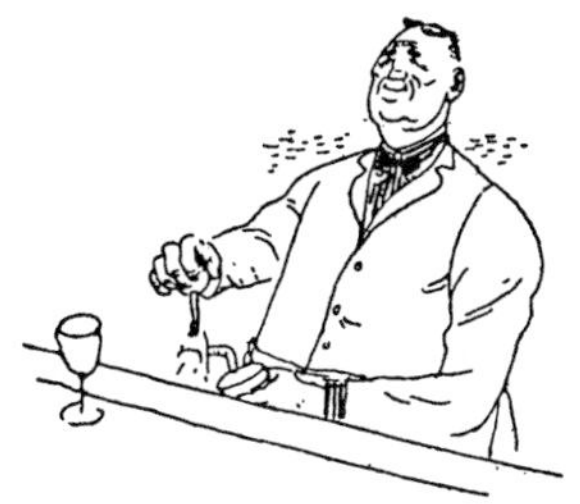

ulcer." She had "argyrosis" — silver deposited in the flesh and tarnished. That was a near miss for me. But let her remain in our sideshow. In real sideshows, they are common. They are billed as the "Blue Boys."

Make way for another exhibit. A Belgian, yellow, frightened. From top to bottom, a nice bright orange. "Yellow jaundice," he called it, just as though there might be several varieties, which there are not. He was convinced he had cancer — cancer of the liver. A neighbor had told him, "Jaundice always goes with liver cancer." This may be nearly true, but the reverse is not the case. Cancer does not always accompany jaundice. Besides he didn't have jaundice. It was springtime and, to get his mind off his imagined tragedy, I inquired, "What have you in your garden?" "Everything, Doctor," he beamed. "The carrots are prime right now, sweet and tender as a mushmelon. Every night I eat a 'bait'; in the morning I have fried carrots. Eat them when they're young is my ticket. Soon enough, they'll be tough." Well and good, the diagnosis is made — "carrotinemia." The yellow pigment of the carrots taken in large "baits" has gotten into his blood and his skin. Harmless indeed. He doesn't even have to stop eating carrots.

A new arrival in the social swirl, needlessly was covering up his years of toil as a coal miner. Yet on his forehead was a headlight of proof. A tenuous scar unmistakably was a clear greenish-blue. This is the telltale powder burn scar. Of course, he might have acquired this blasting stumps or setting off fireworks. Denying his honest "trademark" is not impressive; evidence is to the contrary. That is why he is added to our galaxy for the sideshow.

Advance word gave notice that a patient with an unnusual nervous disease soon would put in appearance. He did. As he walked in, his face was expressionless as any doll. He might have been wearing a "dough face," ready for a mummer's parade. Walking the twenty feet from the door to my desk, he bumped into the desk's edge with the impact of a blind man's misstep. He was not blind. My examination was over, diagnosis made. The patient in ten seconds demonstrated his affliction — manganese poisoning. "What did he reveal so quickly?" Mask-like facies and propulsion — inability to stop when walking. Of course, I had to prove exposure. There was abundant exposure to manganese dusts.

Eschewing fingerprints as trite stuff, our pursuit of trade detection has provided a group of fingernail color clues. Women are banned from the line-up since their nails already may be colored. If the nails are black (not dirty) make your first choice "mercury worker"; if yellow, picric acid, or TNT, or nitric acid. If nails distinctly are purplish, suspect the chemical worker; if brown, we have a wider choice, such as from chromates, photographers' baths, or potassium manganese soaks for infections. Ashen blue nails belong to the silver worker or the silver taker. My own right hand nails acquired a deep brown color, to my consternation. Like everything else, the cause came out. An innocent looking hair tonic had been doctored a bit by its manufacturer — feeling perhaps, that while most persons would scorn to purchase a known hair dye, these same persons would rejoice in the return of natural hair color. My hair remained white, but my nails like the dye. I, with my tonsorial stigmata, take a place alongside the others in the sideshow.

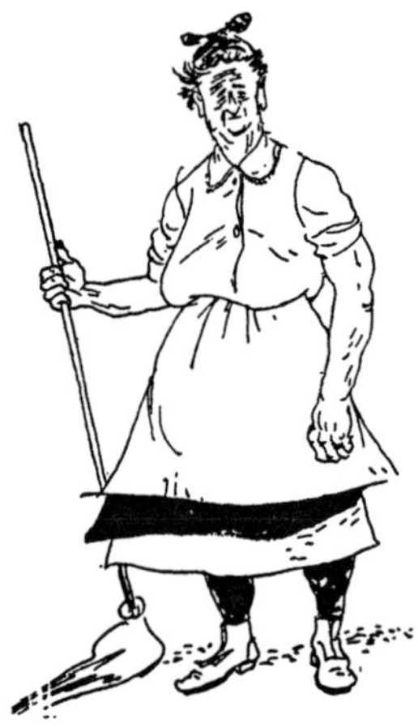

The only possible justification for inclusion of "cauliflower ears" as the "trademark" of the pugilist stems from the belief that all of us enjoy reading those things about which we know much already. For our purposes, I am not displaying any pugilist with his proof of his opponent's skill. Always a step ahead is requisite. So please note that military tank crewmen are the newest additions to that large group of task performers who may advertise their jobs by physical indications.

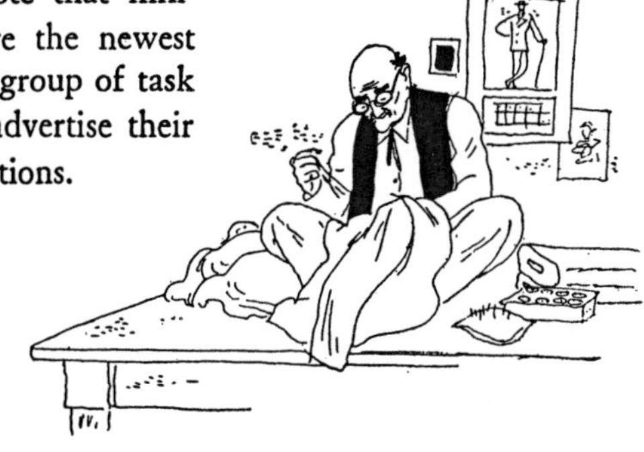

Take a look at the man in the booth next to the last. He is pitted and scarred, over his chest, face, and legs. The scars are small and there are many of them. A lot of brown pigment surrounds the whitish scars. Do your own labeling as to his job. You can't fail. That's correct. He is a foundryman. His scars are from splashed molten metal.

By their corns, ye shall know them. A hundred trades may introduce themselves by their favorite site for a callus. Before the main show resumes there is time only for six. If the corns are grooved skin thickenings, on the outside of the little finger — it's the bundle wrapper. Wrapping string is the cause. If the calluses are on the shoulders — it's the hod carrier. If the skin thickening is over the abdomen, it could be on a bartender or at least someone who continually rubs against the counter edge. If on the lips, a corn marks the wind instrument musician. If on the inner surface of the forearm and in a woman, you probably are dealing with an old-time washwoman. If on the inner surface of the thumb and at the same time front and back of all other fingers, you probably have a tailor on your hands — a hand cutter — these are corns from shears.

It is an ancient custom among us pitchmen, never to have more than fifteen attractions in the sideshow for fear of detraction from the main show. So, having reached fifteen, may I ask that you in your goodwill pass right through the page into the main tent.

Chapter 21

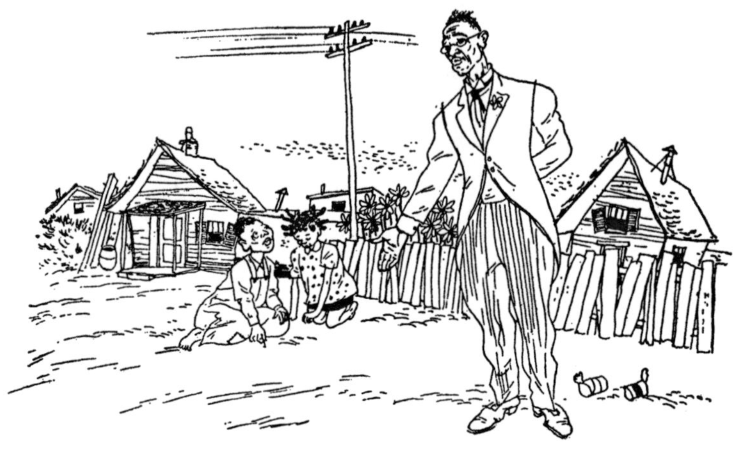

The Tale of Two Coats

THE PLANT where "Rafe" worked would have been praised if described as a "sweat shop." Work here, in the parlance of laborers, was a "last chance job." Tow sacks, burlap bags and "gunnies" discarded by industry, thrown out by markets, picked up in gutters and alleys, were given a semblance of cleaning in this factory, were shredded by machines and the coarse fibered product brought together as jute battings. In time, these shabby pads find their way into cheaply upholstered furniture where gaudy coverings hide the unsightly mess beneath.

No industrial operation could have been made much more dusty. The law of the state required that the shredding machinery should be fitted with a dust collector and fan, but this inadequate law failed to specify that the collected dust should be transported to some non-dangerous area. The vicious employer, worthy of no consideration, evaded the protective purposes of the law by installing the prescribed hood and blower, but conducting the accumulated dust for only a few feet and then discharging it in the open air of the same room. To conserve the public health, it was necessary to prosecute this recalcitrant employer, preying upon the vitals of his few employees. Rafe was Exhibit A.

No x-ray of the chest was needed to mark this negro as probably having tuberculosis. Shiny-eyed, emaciated, languid—even when covered with dust Rafe presented that "general appearance" of tuberculosis so obvious to the physician.

Later the x-ray report came to hand, but its contents had been anticipated. It read, "Moderately advanced tuberculosis, bilateral. This patient should be hospitalized."

It became my duty to tell Rafe that he might not do any further work. At first only casually and gently it was suggested to Rafe that it might not be good for him. He didn't agree.

"I ain't feelin' rat peart. Th' dust at the works gits in my throat, but I reckon I cain't complain."

Trying to gain Rafe's confidence, I inquired, "Where were you born?"

"Down in Alabama, out a piece from Hanceville."

I observed that I too was born in Alabama, but not near Hanceville.

"Anyway," said Rafe, "you is my frien'."

"Of course I'm your friend, and in your sickness you're going to need a lot of friendship."

The negro is slow to confide in the white man, but our shared state of birth impelled Rafe to an eager burst of confidence.

"If you is my frien', then I can tell you that I'se a po't, a verse maker, a po'try song maker."

"Maybe in the hospital you'll have plenty of time for writing poetry."

"Sho will, Doctor, and I'll write some pretty po'tries about you."

It is the way of hospitals seldom to be in a hurry save in the presence of emergencies, so three weeks elapsed before Rafe was called in as a patient. In the meantime, he who should have been continuously in bed was not idle.

One Sunday morning, seated in the garden, I noticed a parting of the shrubbery and there was Rafe. He was excited, anxious.

"Doctor," he said, "somethin's happened!"

My guess was that he was going to tell me that he had had a pulmonary hemorrhage the night before. He didn't.

"Doctor, I been made Pres'dent of the International 'Ciety of Cullud Gen'uses, Po'ts and Musicians."

"Splendid, Rafe."

"An' that ain' all. We's havin' our ann'al meetin' rat here in this here town today."

"Where you going to have the meeting? In one of the churches?"

"No suh, they's a vacant lot rat by my house with grass and some trees. We's goin' to have th' meetin' there. This is my big chance, Doctor."

"How did you get to be President of the Society."

"Doctor, I 'lected myself. You see I organized the 'Ciety of us Gen'uses, Po'ts and Musicians."

"Are there any other officers?"

"Yes suh. There's plenty of officers. Vice pres'dents, secretaries, trustees, but ah'm all of them, too. Would you like to hear some of my po'try? I'll say some and sing some if you'll let me."

I dreaded this ordeal. I need not have. With a quality a little akin to Stephen Foster, Rafe had made songs of genuine beauty. In his own soft Alabama voice, plus the inspiration of some invisible urge in this doomed man, Rafe poured out a beauty of words in keeping with the beauty of the garden where he stood. Finishing his songs, he got around to the real reason for his visit.

"I got to make all of them folks know that I is the best po'm maker of them all, an' the best musician. I'm goin' to sing them songs and tell them verses that I made up 'til they know that they done right in making me Pres'dent of the 'Ciety. But I cain't do it lessen one thing happens. I got to have clothes like a gen'us oughta have. Once't at a party where I waited on table, I seen you there in a long coat and striped pants. All night long I been prayin' to God tellin' him I wondered if I got them clothes all nice and cleaned up afterwards, if you'd let me wear your long coat and striped pants when I 'dresses the other gen'uses, po'ts and musicians today."

Poor starved life, threadbare of all the things his soul longed for — these clothes were the ultimate in happiness for him — success, fame, everything.

Rafe got the suit, a wing collar, grey tie, and cuff links.

On that Sunday afternoon drive, I found myself headed toward Rafe's part of the village. I wanted to see the assembled "geniuses, poets and musicians." Maybe I just wanted to see my suit on Rafe. My only hesitancy was a dread of a traffic jam on Rafe's narrow street. This hazard I risked.

As we neared the house, there was not a car or a person in sight. Over beyond the house where the lawn was, stood Rafe, addressing the assembled "International Colored Geniuses." His audience consisted of two negro children, about ten years old — a boy and a girl, sitting on the ground. They were poking long green stalks of daffodils down into wormholes in the earth, hoping that some unwary worm might take hold and be snapped out. No whit of attention did they pay to Rafe. But this was not impolite. Rafe with his shining eyes, in total fantasy was addressing an imaginary audience of thousands of his people.

A few days later Rafe went to the hospital. Once weekly his wife, with some of her five children, came to the back door and brought us word of Rafe's condition.

At first her news was good.

"Rafe's got a rat nice place to be sick in. The doctors see him ever' day. White nurses takes care of him. Sometimes he is on the po'ch, and sometimes he is in the big inside room. Rafe just lies there and makes new po'try. You kin see his lips movin', but the doctor won't let him write it down on paper. They say he's too weak."

In time the word brought by Georgia Belle was not reassuring.

"Looks like Rafe's goin' to die. Sometimes he don' even know me. He talks a lot, but it ain't pretty po'try no more."

Rafe did die. On a Saturday morning, Georgia Belle with all of her five little girls stood at the back door with her ill news. There was something a bit proud and defiant in Georgia Belle's demeanor — something that scarcely fitted this occasion, of this lowly negress with her dead husband.

"Doctor," she said, "won't you set out in the yard and let me talk about somepin' 'at's botherin' me?"

We went to the garden. Georgia Belle did all the talking for the family.

"I'm the widow of the greatest cullud po't in the world and the Pres'dent of the 'Ciety of Cullud Gen'uses, Po'ts and Musicians. I oughta be able to give Rafe a big funeral, but all the money I got is sixty-five cents. At the hospital they told me that the Government would bury Rafe. I wanta ast you if that means that ever'body knows that Rafe was the greatest po't in the world and because of that the Government is goin' to give him a funeral like Abraham Lincoln or the Governor when he died? That sho would be fine if that's what they's countin' on doin'."

I explained to Georgia Belle that, since she had no money, the Government would step in and give Rafe a simple burial, but it would not be like the Governor's.

"But that won't do for Rafe — he was too smart a man. All the folks in this country oughta pitch in and give Rafe the biggest kinda funeral."

Then it was I inquired of Georgia Belle what sort of funeral she would like. To her it was all clear.

"I want a big lot of folks, a grey coffin with white silk linin' an' lots of flowers, an' a cullud preacher who could talk about Rafe. Then," she said, "mostest of all I'd like to drive up to that funeral with all these chillun not in an automobile, but in a big carriage with two horses. Down in Alabama whenever the white folks had a big funeral, they all drove up in carriages."

"But, Georgia Belle," I said, "in this day and time there aren't any carriages. Automobiles are better. What you are suggesting is almost impossible."

Georgia Belle protested that if the world knew how great a poet Rafe had been they would see to it that his widow got to his funeral in a carriage.

The spell of Rafe's simple poetry and the melody of his lays as I had heard them in this same garden were still upon me. I knew then that Rafe was going to have a little better funeral than was in prospect for him. I even hoped that the widow might satisfy her soul through the agency of a two-horse carriage. The family went away with an injunction to return in three hours.

I called my friend, the superintendent of the Tuberculosis Hospital. We had been together in the Army. I knew that any requested favor within reason would be granted, but the request I was about to make was not reasonable.

"Tom," I said," out in your morgue you have the body of a negro named Raphael Tucker."

"Yes."

"What are you going to do with him?"

"Since his family can't bury him, the county will have to do that. We're allowed twenty-five dollars. We'll put him in a pine box and bury him over in the pauper's lot on the hospital property."

"Will there be any funeral service?"

"Not unless the family is around or any of his friends. Then the colored chaplain might hold a little service."

"Tom, in this case, you're going to do nothing of the sort. For once you are going to do something very fine."

The story of Rafe was told — the story of the International Society of Colored Geniuses, Poets and Musicians, the story of Rafe's songs and poems, the story of Rafe's proud, adoring wife.

"Let's do something for this colored boy in death. The world has done nothing but pick on him in life. Let's give him a funeral."

Dr. Tom quickly and gladly fell in with the plan.

"Here's how it can be managed. By luck tomorrow is colored Sunday. Once every month we have colored religious services in the chapel on Sunday afternoon. If there has been a death among the colored patients, we ordinarily build the services around a funeral. The negro visitors prefer that sort of service. There will be three or four hundred out tomorrow afternoon, and we'll have the negro's funeral in the big chapel."

"What about a preacher?"

"There will be a half dozen in the crowd. We'll have them all to sit on the platform. I know them all. We'll have a fine service about poets and poetry and it will be very sincere."

"But," I said, "you can't take a plain pine box and make it fit into this elaborate ceremony."

"That can be managed too. The undertakers' association keeps out here at the hospital a small assortment of caskets as samples. The families of dead patients frequently make their selection right here on the grounds and this is convenient for the undertakers. The caskets now on hand are showing a little wear, and the plan is to call them in and send out a new lot. We'll just borrow one of these old caskets which are plenty good."

"Has he got any clothes in which to be buried?"

"That doesn't matter. We're going to have him at his funeral service dressed up in evening clothes. At the hospital we have a dramatic club and in its wardrobe are all sorts of costumes, suits, and other garments. These are used over and over and are recleaned. We will dress your poet better than he ever was in life."

"Could you rustle a little music?"

"That's settled. Among the visiting negro groups are several choirs who go about the wards singing to the patients. At least one choir and a soloist will participate. Leave all that to me."

To this medical superintendent I was Major, and so he addressed me, saying, "Major, what I'm going to do is all set, but you've got to get a two-horse carriage for the widow. That's your job. Have her and the children over here in the carriage Sunday afternoon at

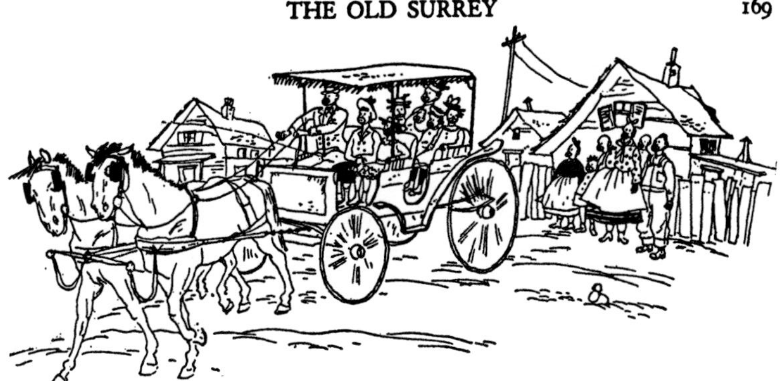

three o'clock, for her poet is going to be honored. You and I may be a little crooked, but in her eyes he is going to be given recognition."

My neighbor on the hill had an old surrey in his barn. Only once had I seen it, and that was at the time of a barn costume party. With two spanking farm horses hitched to this carriage, he and his family had driven to the dance. Now my eyes were on this outfit.

"Carlos, have you still got that old surrey in your barn?"

"Yes, but it hasn't been out for years and years. I guess I ought to throw the old contraption away."

"Not until after tomorrow."

"What's going on?"

He too heard the story of the colored genius, his songs, his woes.

"Sure," he said, "we can fix it up. It's about five miles over to the hospital. We'd better allow about two hours. I'll get Oscar to put on his old coachman's outfit and his high hat. He actually drove the carriages on the place about thirty-five years ago. He'll be at your negro's home tomorrow afternoon at one o'clock."

That Sunday afternoon in the little chapel of the hospital, there were row after row of solemn-faced negroes, whose love of solemnity, of things emotional, had brought them there. Some knew Rafe; more did not, but with one accord they were all prepared to lift their voices in a murmuring chant of praise, or a piercing shriek ending in a wailing crescendo. "Yes, Lawdy, yes, Jesus, have mercy."

The voice of the soloist rose clear and strong above the others, keenly aware of its power to sway them —

"Nothing between my soul and my Saviour; naught of this world's delusive dreams."

Now the negro minister spoke, his intelligent voice rising in eulogy of Rafe. There were flowers and music and the silk-lined casket, its bright handles gleaming in the afternoon light — things on a higher scale than Rafe had known in life, but for which his heart had reached. When it was over, Georgia Belle, with her head lifted high, her face full of glory, came to me.

"Doctor, it was grand. I always thought folks knew there wasn't nobody smarter'n Rafe. They sent us that big carriage with those two horses, th' man in th' blue coat and yellow pants to drive th' horses. Ever'body in th' cullud part of town come to see us drive off, an' all them as could, come to th' funeral. There musta been ten thousand folks there. Th' preacher made a pretty talk about Rafe an' Lawdy, Doctor, that coffin musta cost five hundred dollars. An' th' clothes he had on, jus' like Rafe always wanted! Now they done tole us jus' to go on home, that they'll take ker of th' buryin' — co'se we don't do that way down home in Alabama — we allus see our dead to their las' restin' place, but I guess with a man as smart as Rafe, an' knowed by all these folks — " Her voice drifted off in wonderment at the miracles of fame.

Later, when I called the hospital superintendent, his account was more dispassionate. "We gave your poet a big funeral service, but after we sent them away we had to put the body in the county's standard pine box and we buried him in the paupers' graveyard. You and I probably will go to hell for this."

But I wasn't thinking of hell or heaven just then, rather of our sorry world where sometimes, if we are to be humans as well as doctors, being crooked like this seems not at all wrong. Honest or dishonest, cupidus or sincere, pretense or reality, the scheme had worked — the gesture had been made of making amends to this colored boy who did, in truth, possess some flame of genius.

Chapter 22

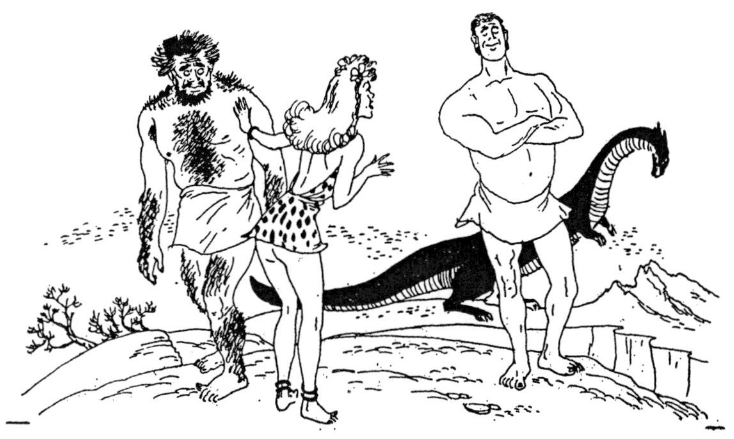

Saving the Surface

WHEN MAN's predecessor, a million years ago, reached the decision to go down through the ages in stark and disgraceful nakedness, he may have overlooked the fact that he was paving the way for trouble for his descendants who would run around in factories instead of tree-tops.

Scantiness of hair may have been accepted by the amorously disposed as such a mark of beauty that the shaggy coated ones found themselves pushed aside into extinction. More likely it is that abundance of food in some favorable eon built up such a thick layer of subcutaneous fat that the protection of hair for warmth became unnecessary. In any conclave of the world's animals meeting as peers and speaking a common language, man's nakedness probably would excite laughter, curiosity, and pity. The embarrassed seating committee would locate man on the back row with the porcupine on his right and the duckbilled platypus on his left. All monstrosities.

Whatever may have been the cause of man's indecent, unhirsuted state, it makes the industrial worker more vulnerable to occupational skin diseases than any other that might befall. The number of skin cases is more than double all other occupational diseases combined, and the number of work materials that may injure the skin may be tenfold the aggregate of substances disturbing only to other portions of the body.

Possibly in an attempt at apology for the blunder of nakedness of mankind, nature makes some of her children dark skinned or black. Shared by every physician is the knowledge that the brunette, the negro, the Mexican, the Japanese, may go about duties handling skin-harmful substances with far less prospect of a dermatitis than the blonde or redhead. The albino-like towhead who has to work like the rest of us oftentimes is as handicapped as some other worker with three fingers off the right hand.

Three hundred thousand workers yearly muddle up their full capacity for work through the acquisition of some occupational dermatosis, but fortunately, uncomplicated, no industrial dermatitis is likely to result in death.

For the physician, these annoying if not always disabling skin diseases may be doubly troublesome. Exact causes of dermatoses are determined only with difficulty, and certainty that they are of work origin or aggravation often is lacking. Most systemic occupational diseases, such as from benzol, carbon tetrachloride, or silica are near precise entities. They make a pathologic blueprint of themselves in apparent willingness to be recognized by a physician. Not so with dermatitis. The rash from industrially-used naphtha with fair fidelity may resemble the dermatitis from the soap used at home or from the turpentine used in paint applied to the hen house. So numerous are the causes of industrial skin diseases and so well is this fact known to workers that, to the mind of almost every worker, any skin disease naturally is laid to his work materials and his employer's responsibility. Not always is this right, or fair.

In one plant where enameled stove-ware was made, there came into the plant dispensary a belligerent workman. Here and there over his arms, legs, and torso were splotches of skin disease, but wholly unlike the customary acute dermatitis produced by work irritants.

"Doc, I wish you'd look me over a little. This has been coming on for two or three days. I don't know as I can work, with this getting worse all the time. Looks like the enamel that I spray with finally got in its licks. Been working with this eight years before and nothing ever happened, but I guess my time's come. Will you make out some papers for me so that I can get insurance?"

The knowing doctor went about his examination in silence. Clearly this workman was the unproud owner of a troublesome skin affair, but the doctor knew that nothing in the liquid enamel might cause this type of lesion, and if it might have, the damage would be to the exposed hands, probably the neck and face—least likely of all might the injured areas appear on the torso.

The doctor had a job to do. Here was a workman fully self-convinced that his skin disease must have resulted from his work and that in nowise was he responsible for its causation or its care. On the other hand, here was a physician, professionally sure that work played no iota of influence. The doctor had seen this peculiar type of skin disease before and knew its cause, but how to spring this unfavorable decision on the workman and still retain his good will for the medical department and his employer was the problem. He decided to do it boldly.

"Jake, I'm going to play magician with you. At home you have been taking some medicine. You have been taking this for a good long while—maybe three or four weeks. You've been taking this medicine because you're constipated—your bowels wouldn't move. What is it you have been taking?"

"How'd you know that, Doc? I never brought any of that medicine to the factory, and I never told any of the boys. Is my mouth brown?"

Then Jake named a much-advertised laxative which is known by every physician to contain phenolphthalein. Only phenolphthalein can produce the peculiar qualities that marked Jake's skin disease.

"Jake, if you'll stop taking that patent medicine, your skin disease will go away — that's what's causing it. You won't have to lose any time, and it isn't going to get any worse if you stop drugging yourself. You may need a laxative, but there are lots better ones than those that contain the drug you're using. Just to prove that the enamel isn't to blame, I want you to go ahead with your work, stop your drug, but come back here a week or ten days from now and I'll make you a present of a package of cigarettes if all your skin disease hasn't gone or isn't going fast."

That is the sort of problem that makes old men out of plant physicians. Name any dozen trades. For half of them I will name some associated material or practice that may damage the skin sur-

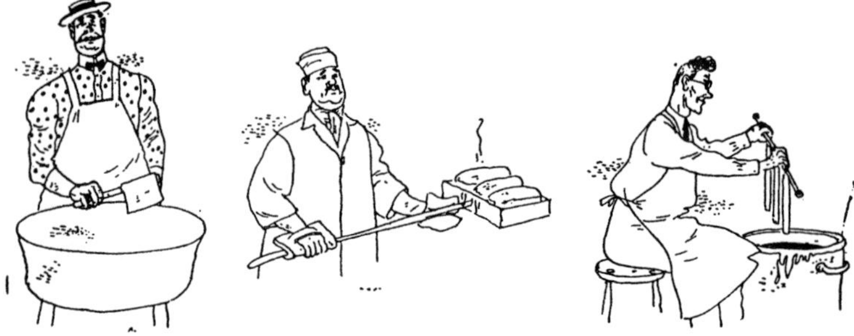

face. If you name the "butcher, the baker, the candlestick maker" in facetious compliance with my overture, I in utter seriousness will describe one of the well-known skin diseases of these three tradesmen, and this I do.

Among all butchers, fish and poultry dealers, meat cooks and game handlers, there is a fair frequency of an acute skin disease called erysipeloid.

This same condition is known among pearl button carvers who cut buttons from mussel shell, at times none too free from decomposing clam flesh.

The baker, like the butcher, is subject to at least half a dozen skin diseases, chief of which are caused by the bleaching agents introduced into flours so that they approach snow-whiteness.

The candlestick maker owes his best known dermatitis to paraffin. Not all candles are made from paraffin, but wherever this substance is manipulated, paraffin boils are possible.

For most of us the symbols of industry are whirring machines, conveyor belts, assembly lines, flowing chemicals. It is easier to associate skin disease with this form of industry, but consider instead the theater's orchestra as an aggregation of workmen. Look at the left collarbone region of the violin player and find there the thickened, horny, overused skin. This is his particular occupational dermatosis and the tell-tale marking of his profession. Then turn to the harpist. His mark of years of playing and practice may be found in the corns on his fingertips.

In the presence of suspected industrial dermatitis, it is not always easy to spot the exact offending chemical in the complex mixtures that now characterize industry's liquids.

Forty years ago paint could be trusted to contain little else in the way of fluids than linseed oil and turpentine. Today a paint formula may put to shame a physician's shotgun prescription. Twelve ingredients — which one is the troublemaker?

In a large factory, there was entrusted to me a troublesome epidemic of nearly two hundred cases of an obvious industrial dermatitis. The workers involved were machinists. All were exposed to oil, cutting compounds, "soda water," steel slivers. The cutting oils had been treated with a disinfectant to lessen the oil's bacterial content. What was the cause?

Already this plant had installed and operated centrifuges to throw out the metal particles. Already too the corporation had installed a pasteurizing unit to treat the oil. Still the epidemic spread. Nearly every workman had his own theory as to where the blame lay. Some jumpy ones were quite sure that a few syphilitics were among them, and that they were spreading the disease. This, of course, was unlikely. Others were convinced that a part of the men were using the oil troughs as urinals, which act unfortunately does happen in low-grade machine shops. Still others decided that within their number there were those who must be suffering from "athlete's foot," and that the fungi from these toes in some manner were being spread throughout the plant.

After treating the more afflicted ones, and attempting to allay the apprehensions of all, I set about the task of determining the real cause. It proved to be no great task. The washroom in this department had been removed to a far corner of the plant, a block away, in order to make room for new machinery. The machinists, a little resentful and a little lazy, resorted to washing up in buckets of gasoline which were hidden about their machines, under benches and in dark corners. Gasoline, much used as it is, in contact with begrimed skin is quite capable of both defatting and irritating human skin. This was the cause of the epidemic.

In almost every group of occupational diseases, there is some key procedure essential to diagnosis. In dusty lung diseases this key is the x-ray. In lead poisoning, the key is the quantitative determination of lead in urine or blood. In the case of occupational skin diseases, the corresponding key is the patch test. In a given lacquer there may be as many as twenty different constituents, including cellulose, ester gum, Damar gum, zinc stearate, zinc sulfide, zinc oxide, titanium dioxide, various alcohols, divers acetates, raw and blown castor oil, toluol, zylol, and naphtha.

In the presence of a recurring dermatitis in a lacquer worker, it may be highly desirable to know precisely what ingredient is responsible. If the physician is contented to make a diagnosis of "lacquer dermatitis," this is cruel to the workman, since practically it sentences him to eliminate himself from the entire paint manufacturing industry, as many of these ingredients are common to scores of coating products. If an exact determination may be made as to the particular constituent offensive to the skin of that workman, then he may be retained in industry so long as he works on products free of that particular substance.

To establish this, minute quantities and always below the amount likely to irritate normal skin, are applied to some uninvolved portion of the workman's skin, usually the back. It is possible to apply a score of these tests at a time. These several test materials are carefully segregated one from another by being kept in place by small squares of gauze overlying rubber damming and adhesive. Oftentimes, but not always, the skin will be irritated by some one and only one of these test substances. After the patch tests have been worn for from six to forty-eight hours, depending upon the judgment of the physician, they are removed and a single inflamed area may reveal the sole agent for which the skin has developed a pathologic distaste. Thus an exact diagnosis has been made.

In the intervening time between the first and last drafts of this chapter, more than 900 patch tests have been applied to my own back, arms, and legs. Why? I don't have up to this moment any skin disease, but some human must be the victim for tests on the hundreds of new materials before their entry into industry. Guinea pigs and rabbits may not be suitably responsive. "Do they hurt? Do I get blisters? Does my skin peel off?" "Yes" to all, but what of it? In some far-off day, I hope, when I shall have developed a universal sensitivity and I am no longer as good even as the rabbits, I shall say in the midst of scratching — "My old skin not only has served me uncommonly well, but in addition, has served a million workers." That may justify the scabs, should I offend you.

Chapter 23

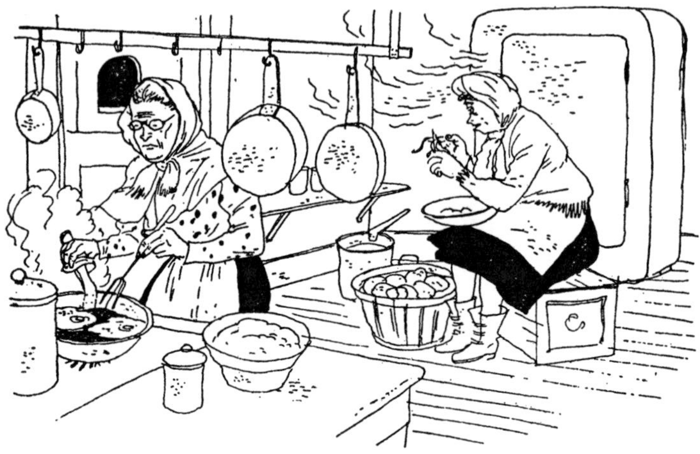

Threats from the Refrigerator

MY INVESTIGATION of dangerous work materials frequently has been characterized by surges limited to one particular substance, or groups of substances closely akin. For years I did little save investigations of dust exposures. At various times there have been surges connected with lead poisoning, in different industries. One entire year was given over to inquiries into the dangers of chlorinated hydrocarbons, chiefly carbon tetrachloride.

At one time I was typed as being especially qualified in regard to refrigerants, methyl chloride, ammonia, sulfur dioxide. While inclination and specialization would have kept me in the factories where mechanical refrigerators were produced, calls for my services, pleasing to relate, arose when disaster followed the defects of refrigerator systems in homes, apartment houses, and other buildings. A single tale will earmark my participation.

In December, 1931, there came to my office from a coal mining town in West Virginia, Mrs. Laval, a patient scarcely able to travel, but with an eagerness to relate an engaging medical story.

In some of the coal mining camps, there are no hotels, nor adequate places for unmarried coal mine workers to live or to house non-resident executives during their visits to the mine sites. This has led to the operation by the mining companies themselves of "clubs."

These clubs provide accommodations for all persons sponsored by the mining company, but permit the right to exclude those persons regarded as undesirable. It was Mrs. Laval's job to operate one mining company's "club." Her duties were those of any manager of a small hotel.

Being an enterprising company, a mechanical refrigerator was installed, replacing an outmoded ice-box. For six months, everyone was delighted — the kitchen help, the serving maids; but chiefly Mrs. Laval was proud of the improvement in her kitchen. Then the refrigerator began to leak irritating gases. Mrs. Laval and all her help, she related, began to cough and sneeze continuously. This was accompanied by nausea, irritation of the eyes and throat. Complaints were made to the management but these complaints were laughed at as being imaginary. So much gas was present that during the winter it was necessary to work with all doors and windows open, thus replacing a portion of the exposure to gases with exposure to cold. All the kitchen and pantry workers went about their duties in winter coats, sweaters, head coverings, and sometimes even with gloves. Mrs. Laval's own work table in the large kitchen, unhappily, was located closest to the refrigerator.

As a result of many complaints, a refrigerator repairman in time made his way up the mountains in the spring of 1930 to repair the leak that no one apart from the kitchen force was willing to believe existed until the refrigerator lost its chilling properties. This repairman furnished two pieces of information, or better one piece of information which later became helpful in making diagnoses and a piece of misinformation, which possibly was responsible for the major disaster. This repairman pointed out that he was charging the refrigerator with thirty pounds of liquid sulphur dioxide and nine pounds of liquid methyl chloride. Both of these gases are decidedly toxic when exposure is extensive. The misinformation came when he scoffed at the possibility of any damage from either of these gases.

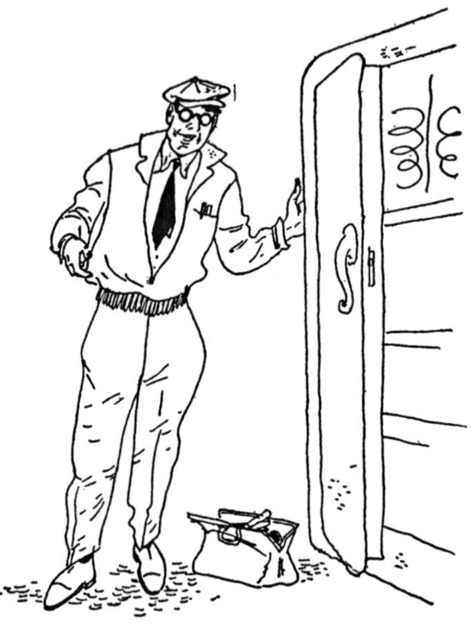

"Why, these gases are used by doctors in the treatment of all sorts of 'bronical' trouble. All you women around here have nothing but winter colds. If there ever should be another leak in the refrigerator system, you ought to get down over the leak with a blanket or a shawl over your head and breathe in these gases for medicine."

For five days the refrigerator operated in proper fashion and then the leak returned — worse than ever. These afflicted workers now had opportunity, believing the word of the refrigerator man, to "cure their colds." At one time four distressed women huddled over the leaking pipe painfully breathing in gases that they had been led to accept as curative. Mrs. Laval was one of the four.

In the hospital there was a stormy period of pneumonia and bronchitis. Slowly she improved, she related, as she completed her history statements, but "Even now," she pointed out, "I have almost continuous asthma — I'm so short of breath that I'm scarcely able to talk without effort, cough during many spells every day and every night, have not regained my thirty pounds lost weight, and certainly can't do any work. I'm a sick woman. Don't you think that in some way the company ought to make amends for the way it treated me?"

"That," I replied, "must at least await my examination and the examination of other doctors, along with an x-ray of your chest."

Many examinations were carried out. When all reports were in, we made many precise medical diagnoses. Expressing these in non-medical terms, Mrs. Laval was suffering from asthma, a marked chronic bronchitis, congestion and inflammation of her nasal passages and throat, high blood pressure, chronic heart disease, some residual effects of her old pneumonia, together with kidney inflammation.

Added to this was a highly emotional state from worries over her many woes. It was agreed that Mrs. Laval was a sick woman, but at her age of sixty-six, many of her abnormalities might not be laid directly at the door of any toxic gas.

All of these things we reported to Mrs. Laval's attorneys, but I took pains to record the fact that our examinations were carried out more than a year after the last of her exposures and her pneumonia episode. I could not be sure from our findings alone that refrigerator gases produced any or all of the conditions present. With accuracy I did point out that methyl chloride in sufficient quantities could produce unconsciousness and death and had done so in other refrigerator cases, notably in Chicago a few years earlier. I pointed out the highly irritating properties of sulfur dioxide and its capacity to produce bronchitis and inflammation of the lungs, to which pneumonia might be a ready sequence.

A few weeks later there came an invitation to participate in the trial of Mrs. Laval's suit. This I was glad to accept — it meant increased experience, a modest fee and an opportunity to testify in behalf of a woman whose straightforward story of neglect when exposed to dangerous gases carried conviction. Mr. Ludlow, her attorney, in writing me had requested that I bring down numerous books, reprints and all possible records, stating, "In West Virginia, these may be used to a greater extent in court work than in some other states."

In my reply I inquired if it would not be well for me to come down one day prior to the beginning of the hearing for conference purposes. Mr. Ludlow flatteringly declined, stating that I would be well able to take care of myself without any conferences. Of course the real reason was that he wished to avoid my charges for one extra day.

Early in the morning of the trial day, I appeared at the little county-seat town in the West Virginia mountains. Long before the trial hour, I hunted up his office, where a friendly secretary told me that Mr. Ludlow would not come in from his farm until the immediate time of the trial, but that she would like to do for me anything that she could to make my stay pleasant. I was a bit unhappy, because once having attached myself to what I believed to be a meritorious claim, my whole yearning was to win. Rules 1, 2, 3, and on are "to win." If Mr. Ludlow preferred no preliminary conferences, well and good — it was no hair out of my scalp. One minute before the trial was due to start at ten o'clock, in came Mr. Ludlow, whom I had met previously and knew to be young, mentally and physically alert, wise in the ways of his West Virginia mountain people and its corporations.

He said, "Doctor, there will be no objection to your sitting at my side at counsel table. You will not go on the stand until the afternoon. If you have brought books and papers, I want you to lay them out on the table and put out all that you have. There will be many witnesses during the morning, and I want you to write frequent notes to me on scraps of paper and whisper to me frequently."

Being puzzled, I inquired, "But what sort of notes? What shall I whisper?"

His reply still further puzzled me. "It makes no difference at all. Write anything and whisper anything, but do something every few minutes."

Still befuddled, I wrote many inane notes, gravely passing them over to Mr. Ludlow. "This is a good witness." "Do we have lunch together?" "Do you think I'll be able to get away tonight?" "You should introduce more photographs." "Ask this claimant more questions about odors." "Let her play up her own symptoms. She's got plenty of them." Interspersed, I followed instructions with whisperings, "Am I writing enough notes?" "Is this next witness the refrigerator repairman?"

It all seemed quite ridiculous. Mr. Ludlow of course had a plan, but I'm a doctor, not a lawyer, and I could not guess his strategy.

During recess, Mr. Ludlow, who knew everyone in the courtroom by his first name, introduced me to many visitors as the "great expert," who would go on the stand immediately on the resumption of trial, after lunch. He invited all to attend, as though it were to be some performance of Joseph Jefferson or Wallace Beery. To me all of this was a bit distasteful, but I didn't know my lawyer.

At the noon recess, Mr. Ludlow said, "Leave all of your books and papers out, don't hide anything. I'll see that they are watched."

"Won't we need some of them at lunch?" I inquired.

"No, we can't have lunch together. I'm tied up in a conference on another case. When you return at one-thirty you go and sit in the witness chair. You'll be sworn in later. The best place to get lunch is at the Phoenix Cafe. Sorry I can't be with you."

Obediently at one-twenty I took my place in the witness chair, which was somewhat elevated, and readily I could look out over the spectators. The courtroom was already filled. Twice as many attended as during the morning.

In came Mr. Ludlow, self-assured, deliberately stopping here and there to greet newcomers among the spectators. Before he reached counsel table, there was a beckoning finger through an open door into one of the judge's private chambers. I was watching Mr. Ludlow attentively and saw a tiny gleam of satisfaction. Then we waited for many minutes. The trial did not start.

Out came the opposing attorneys arm in arm. The trial was over

— settled. We had won. Pleased with himself, Mr. Ludlow came over to me, still in the witness chair, and apologized.

"I knew they wouldn't go ahead. My whole plan has been to play you up. All those notes and whisperings were merely to attract attention to you. Not having lunch with you and not meeting you this morning was all planned. I wanted these good mountain people to recognize that I hadn't the least misgiving about the trial; the jury's award probably would be the full twenty-five thousand dollars that we asked in our petition, but you can't ever tell about the juries, and all day I have been willing to settle for any fair figure. I knew that when I got back from lunch I'd be buttonholed by my opponent."

"All this is quite all right with me, Mr. Ludlow, but why did you have me sit in the witness chair?"

"Well," he said, "you wrote me that your charges would be higher if you actually took the witness stand. You've taken it, even though you didn't testify. Go ahead and make your charges accordingly. The other side is paying for it anyway."

Chapter 24

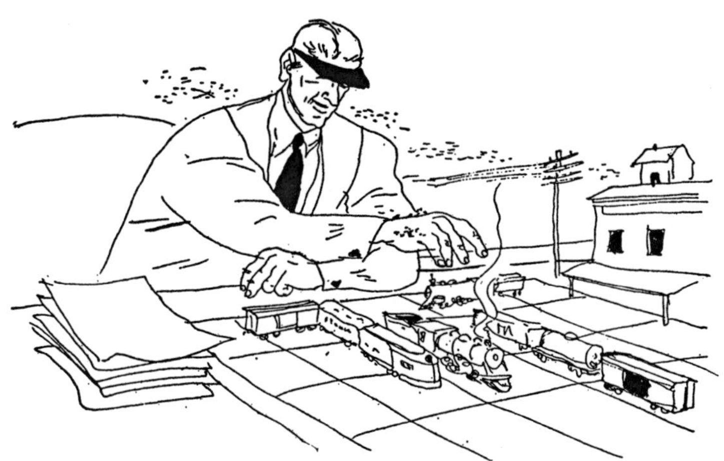

Dancing Eyes

In 1930, the American Train Dispatchers Association, through its able executive, Mr. J. G. Luhrsen, provided for me an outstanding opportunity to investigate the health of train dispatchers. This association president pointed out that within his brotherhood there existed an insurance fund set up and operated on standard actuarial formulae. Under expectations, the insurance premiums charged the association members would have been ample. Actually, continuous drains were made upon the moneys of the insurance fund owing to high death rates and total disabilities. It was the conclusion of this association that unusual work conditions might prove to exist, and might account for the difficulties of the insurance division. I was asked to ascertain the facts.

The train dispatcher is extraordinarily important in train movements. Little known to the public and commonly classed only as a railroad office worker, the dispatcher, to an extent greater than for any other person, is responsible for safety in train operations.

Seated in some office that may be apart from any railroad terminal and out of sight of all trains, the train dispatcher moves his transportation units as so many chessmen on a board. It is the train dispatcher who issues orders to train crews, arranges meeting points, rates of speed, the size of locomotives, the picking up of cars by freight trains, the feeding and watering of stock in transit, the hours of labor of train crews in order to avoid exceeding legal hour limits. At a single time, the train dispatcher may be watching the movements of as many as twenty-five trains. Decisions involving life and death of passengers and crews may on occasion be made at the rate of two hundred per hour, but this is exceptional.

The arrangements made with me called for the careful physical, mental and psychological examination of a large number of train dispatchers with examining points in New York, Newark, Birmingham, Omaha, Cincinnati, Covington and Somerset, Kentucky.

The indulgence of no publisher, however friendly, would permit me to narrate the full story of our caravan as it moved from city to city, setting up temporary offices, making special arrangements for x-ray examinations, laboratory tests, specialists for consultations. In the end, we found many acceptable evidences of extraordinary mental and emotional stresses in the life of the train dispatcher, because of his work responsibilities. These stresses and strains took immeasurable toll from his well-being and comfort, reflected in high rates of heart disease, high blood pressure, mental disturbances, frequently suicide, gastro-intestinal diseases. The entire story would require a volume in itself. Let me content myself with the recital of the unexpected finding of a new occupational disease.

In New York, soon after the beginning of the investigation, every train dispatcher was asked to give us from four to six hours for test purposes. This period was distributed over a series of mental, emotional, and fatigue tests, routine physical examinations of every portion of the body from the scalp to the sole, including examination of the interior of the eyeballs, heart exercise tests, blood pressure in various positions, Wassermann tests, urinalyses, blood counts, audiometer tests for hearing, basal metabolic rate determinations, and x-ray examinations. Some tests were made immediately at the end of the work trick of eight hours, and others just prior to the resumption of work on the following day. Some strictly medical examinations were carried out by Dr. Litwin, the psychological and fatigue tests by Mrs. Leonard Minster. Mr. O. H. Braese represented the Dispatchers' Association and arranged for the steady inflow of examinees, and otherwise provided for the excellent cooperation from the train dispatchers themselves. In that city, the laboratory work was subsidized to divers private clinical laboratories. Various medical technicians took medical histories, kept records, performed minor portions of the physical examinations, such as weight taking. It was my job to act as the coordinator, the final reviewer of data, the appraiser of findings. All of us were very busy, for train dispatchers work on three shifts of eight hours. At the beginning we found ourselves working eighteen hours a day.

About the fifth day, the cautious Dr. Litwin, ophthalmoscope in hand, came in and said, "I think I've found something. I haven't been recording it because I wasn't sure, but now I am sure. When these dispatchers come off their job, half of them at least are showing a definite nystagmus."

That was new. No one in this country had ever described any prevalence of an occupational nystagmus. This disease of the eyes is characterized by slow or rapid jerking or rotating of the eyeballs in their sockets quite apart from any control of their owners. At times the movement may be up and down — on other occasions right and left, and in still others the eyes may move in an arc rather than in a straight line. We were much excited and provided new facilities for better examination — the type of chair used in spinning aviators to test their equilibrium sense — equipment to apply heat and cold to the middle ear organs, since such conditions are known to influence these peculiar changes in the eye.

In England, nystagmus is a common occupational disease, occurring in large numbers among coal miners. Special commissions have been created in the British domain to study nystagmus and to devise means for its prevention and control. Its occurrence has been attributed to many causes, such as carbon monoxide in the mines, poor illumination, inadequate diet, fatigue, but most probable of all is that nystagmus in the British coal miner, working in narrow coal seams, is caused by the necessity of rapid eye movements following the hand pick to the point of impact, thence back to the overhanging roof. In the United States, no such opportunities for nystagmus exist. Coal is in such abundance that two-foot seams are seldom worked. Most mines are electrically lighted. Handwork largely has been displaced by mechanical coal cutters and loaders.

Here then was the prospect of an unexpected professional disease — train dispatchers' nystagmus. But our examinations were too few in number. We must wait. We would wait, but we added to our staff Dr. J. F. Bateman, an able neurologist.

Soon came the puzzle. If these train dispatchers do have nystagmus, from what possible source may it come? Could the gases of train smoke induce this disease? This seemed unlikely because many train dispatchers carry out their duties well away from trains.

By this time we had discovered that train dispatchers wearing continually throughout their work period a phone receiving-set over the left ear often presented a one-sided deafness or, more accurately, partial deafness. Might this explain the peculiar dancing of the eyes? I had to lay low this theory when we met with a small group of train dispatchers who carried out their communications not by phone but by telegraphy. Some of these dispatchers likewise displayed nystagmus. Out went the deafness theory.

All the while the correct answer was before us, but not for a time did we recognize it.

Every train dispatcher uses a train sheet. This varies in size with almost every railroad system, but customarily is a rectangular sheet sometimes as large as three by six feet with hundreds of small lined

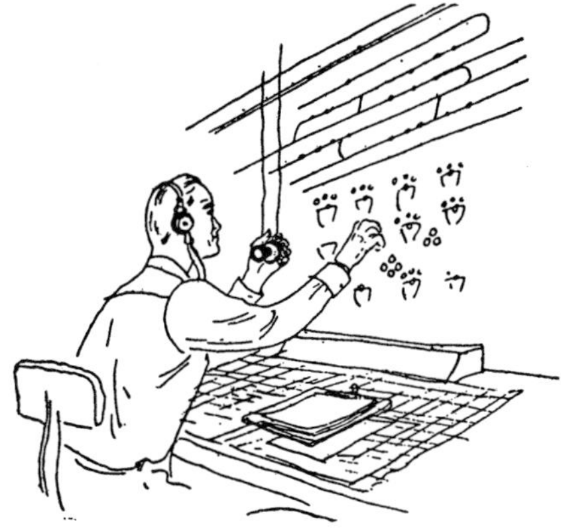

rectangles on both front and back sides. In a left-hand column, every train is entered by the train dispatcher with some notes regarding the crew, physical make-up of the train, etc. To the right are spaces for entry of information from every reporting point. If the dispatcher be operating six or eight trains in each direction, some trains possibly a hundred miles apart may be passing a station every minute. Thus into the ear of the train dispatcher pours endless train information. Every item must be entered, first high up on the page for one train, then at the bottom, then at the extreme right, then perhaps in the center or the left, back again to the bottom.

All the while the train dispatcher's eyes are required quickly to focus on this point and that. His eyes receive no rest. Movement, movement, movement. Here was the answer.

The same old story as in England — the necessity for eye movements in following the motion of the pick and in the train dispatchers the endless motion of the eyes in following the pen in making train entries. In short fatigue, ocular fatigue.

Sixty-seven per cent of all train dispatchers examined were the unwitting owners of these dancing eyes. In train dispatchers, the involuntary movement was right and left, unlike the British coal miners, whose nystagmus usually is circular.

Then came the important decision to be made. How significant is train dispatchers' nystagmus? Should it be regarded as disabling? Would these train dispatchers require two or three years of rest in some instances? Might train wrecks be occasioned by any influence from this disease? How long would the condition persist?

Fortunately all around, it was soon disclosed that train dispatchers' nystagmus is a fleeting affair — one night's rest and the condition often disappeared, only to return by the end of the next work period. In a few cases, the nystagmus continued for at least a week after any exposure, but never were we able to bring together any proof that this unusual movement of the eyes was any more than an evidence of ocular fatigue under peculiar work circumstances. No disability — no chronic form — it was merely the mark of an eye-tired workman.

Chapter 25

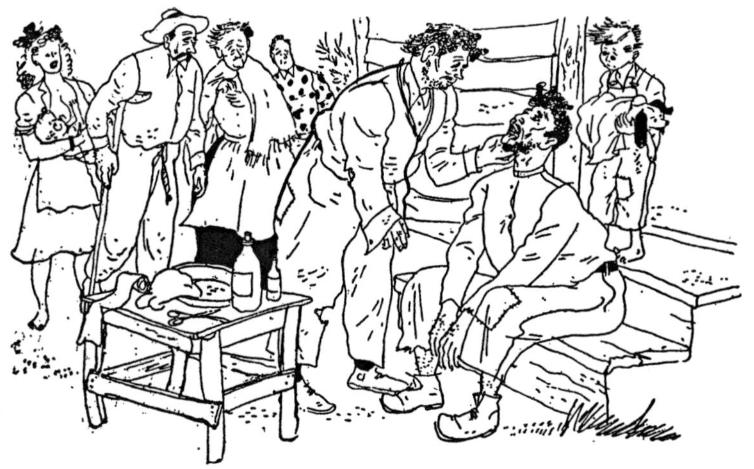

Journey to Junius

WHEN conversation at the dinner table develops a pallor and threatens to fall flat on its face, some hostess-saver is almost sure to toss out some one of the myths about doctors. The conversational pulse at once is strengthened by mention of the fabulous notion that most doctors acquire the disease in which they specialize — the heart specialist develops heart disease — the dermatologist is baldheaded — the psychiatrist goes insane. Denying nothing I only point to the male obstetricians. But wait. Possibly pregnancy is only a physiologic state and not a disease. The myth is saved for the moment.

While all this is going on some diner, in quietly vehement tones that seem to come upward from somewhere around the ankles, is seeking a rehearing for the myth that all doctors are alcoholic. If clever, "ethylic" will be substituted, like the physician dictating in the presence of the patient.

My present drive excludes any concern in the over-all statistics of ethylic doctors. Out of the total I am trying to extricate the saintly Junius for demonstration purposes — not as a physician, not as an alcoholic, not as a saint, but as a patient with an occupational disease. That's Junius' own diagnosis. He, at the end of a losing bout, is apt to bubble: "My occasionally acquired mental recreation through the aid of alcohol is an occupational disease directly the result of my work. I reach the point of not being able to stand any more women talking about the aches, pains, noises, and movements of their bellies."

Since Junius has grafted his disease onto our medical territory, here's his protocol — like all good medical protocols, it starts with childhood.

Fifty-five years ago Junius was a small boy growing up as the sole child in the midst of many adults on a magnificent old plantation in the deep South. Ultra-privileged, he reveled in his own horses and dogs, his personal guns and servants. Spoiled but lovable, he was fitting into the soft life of his forebears.

There were other grandsons and daughters, but none was privileged other than to visit the plantation during the summers. Junius was the unquestioned, unchallenged superior. In simple eagerness, he taught the others to work with dogs over birds, how to fill gun shells, how to saddle a horse, how to swim, where the best muscadines grew, and how to ski on pine straw as a substitute for snow.

Fondly his elders watched his growth into maturity, in full assurance that the family traditions would survive. Then Junius rebelled. He was so foolish as to want to be a doctor. The family acquiesced, but with the covert feeling that, even as a doctor, he still would return to the plantation. After Junius became a doctor, he further outraged the family by professing to wanting to be another Osler, another Welch, or another Marion Simms. He went to New York. It could have been predicted that there too he would be much loved, accepted, successful.

There it was he acquired his "occupational disease." Down, down,

down went Junius. Soon scorned by friends, berated by his wife, crazed by alcohol, Junius disappeared — back to his old South state, but not to his home — not even alcohol could take away that much pride.

Through well-planned calculations, Junius hunted out the most inaccessible, the most forlorn, the most benighted region of the state. Tattered, torn, poverty-stricken and dipsomaniacal, Junius started the practice of medicine, taking few fees, having no home, maintaining no office — the sainthood began.

Some physicians heal by their mere presence, by the laying on of hands, through the assurance of words. This capacity was Junius' chief armamentarium, although from the wreckage of his former greatness he salvaged a few instruments and appliances. Word of miracles spreads rapidly. No publicity agents are required.

Alternately, for weeks at a time, Junius was drunkenly sprawled in some back brushman's house and then, the stupor passed, a performer of wonders. No one questioned his right to drink or chided his excesses. With the passing of the bleariness, Junius would see before him a waiting gathering of hopeful patients. Some lived in temporarily pitched tents, some day by day were driven distances in wagons and buggies and later in automobiles, hoping that on that day sobriety would return.

Like a drunken Christ, Junius walked among them, asking questions, making diagnoses, imparting strength. Foolish it seems that strength might emanate from the sordid mind or body of Junius, but there it was — strength for the sick and the lame. It would be untruthful to make it appear that Junius cured cancer with the touch of his hand or removed brain tumors with his meager equipment. There is sufficient of reality without exaggeration. In his years of sainthood, Junius detected hundreds of cases of pellagra, of parasitic invasions, of malaria, of tuberculosis and others of those conditions for which there are either characteristic treatment regimes or specific cures. Junius, knowing his own limitations, found justification for doing out in the open air a few minor operations with a field hand for first assistant and anesthetist, and with trust in God for sterility.

Those who desired to blame and condemn Junius probably had ample reason. It never occurred to Junius that he was a saint or a worker of miracles. These things did not occur to other physicians in nearby counties, whose practices suffered in proportion to the spreading of Junius' healings.

Word passed around that if one might anticipate the coming of sickness, faithful Junius would stay sober until health had been restored. In practical application, such a proposal limited itself to obstetrics and planned operations. Seekers for the homeless, office-less, car-less Junius needed only to inquire the residence of that woman next most likely to be confined. There Junius would be.

After a silence of twenty years in the euphemistic relationship between doctor and his patient, I set out to beard the Junian scorn for old friendships. Just a professional call on a patient with an "occupational disease," involving twenty-two hundred miles.

Like Johnny Appleseed, Junius had no address, at least no address accessible to the outsider. If Junius' large state were cut into four quarters, many people knew that he might be found in a certain one of those quarters, but where? No roads save mud roads, no telephones, no directories, and, like most saints, Junius was no taxpayer.

In settlement after settlement I made inquiries. Everywhere someone had heard of Junius, but at first the only replies were: "He was here once," or "he is still further South," or "people that come in from the deep brush talk about the old doc a lot."

One day I became "warm." I found, through the rural mail carrier, the pathway that eventually led to Junius. The mail carrier warned me, "If you have any papers to serve on the old doc, you will never get to him. Everyody out there will lie to you, and warn him to get out of sight. If you mean any harm at all, it will do you no good to hunt him. He never can be found unless his friends believe you mean him well. Even the sheriff when he has some papers to serve on him always sends the old doc word two or three days ahead of time and the doc moves on — if he's sober, and you will never get to him. Everybody out there will lie to you, and if he isn't sober, friends tote him around and hide him.

"The folks out there believe that he is a better doctor drunk than most doctors are sober. It's thirty-five miles out in the brush, but if you're bent on going, I'll tell you how to get to a man's house who will take you there."

Many mudholes later, I reached the house of "the man" who knew where Junius might be found. This man looked me over gravely, and in wide-eyed innocence declared that he had never heard of any such person. I protested my fondness for Junius, my plans to serve him well, my professional kinship; the man only shook his head. I played my trump ace, finally.

"You do know all right. You're only protecting him because you think I'm after him. He stayed right here in this house for five weeks before your baby was born two months ago. The old doctor was drunk almost up to the day of your wife's confinement. You spent two weeks trying to sober him up."

The man meekly said, "How did you know that?"

"The mail carrier told me."

"Come on, then," said the man, "I'll take you to him. It's twenty miles away. You've never seen any road like you're going to see now."

Many swamps beyond, and after many local inquiries, we finally stopped in front of a shabby, ramshackle, bedraggled house where Junius was said to be. A little fearful, I said to the man, "Go in and see if he is sober. Tell him I want to see him. Tell him we were boyhood friends."

After a while, the man came out, shaking his head, saying, "He's in there all right and he's sober, but he's been looking out through a crack at you. He says he never saw you before in his life."

Curiosity got the better of Junius for at that moment he opened the door and stood in the doorway. The once magnificent Junius

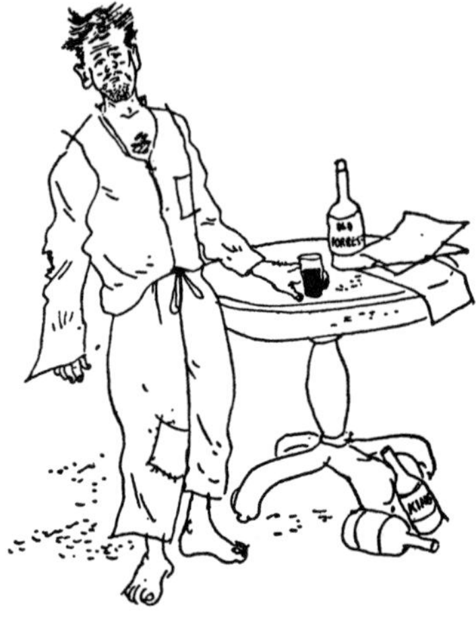

was still magnificent in his tatters. His suit instead of being in rags might be said to be eroded. Later, when I saw his back, a foot square of coat had been cut out to make a new seat for the trousers, probably on the theory that it was more important there.

There stood Junius. The fear was that, in his insecurity, he would quickly close that door and never again would I have access to him. Rushing forward, I shouted, "It's Carey. It's Carey. We grew up together. You know me. You want to see me."

Junius, still magnificent, unbending no whit, gave no evidence of recognition. His greeting after long years was, "While you are in this house, it will not be necessary for you to use your Harvard accent."

I felt rebuked.

I was invited into the temple of the saint, the furnishings of which consisted of a bed, one chair, a washstand with bowl and pitcher. Abashed at Junius' dignity, it seemed best to meet on the common ground of medicine for the moment.

"On the way over," spoke I, hoping for a topic that might be shared, "I saw several cases that suggested avitaminoses."

This touched off Junius. For half an hour, in the purest English Junius poured out an authoritatively scientific lecture on atypical varieties of deficiency diseases. Previously I had thought to present to this tattered offcast of physicians some new word about deficiency diseases. At once I realized I was in the presence of the master. How he acquired this new information, I still do not know. Foolishly I injected one observation that nicotinic acid was being used quite successfully in the treatment of pellagra under some circumstances, and that I had been familiar with this treatment for about a year.

Calmly, and without disdain, Junius observed, "I have been using nicotinic acid for a period of two years."

Again I was put in my place.

In this pause, I leaped into the conversation with a whole series of questions, "Junius, do you remember? Do you recall the time? Have you forgotten?"

I had in mind, and I am sure that he did, a thousand boyhood adventures—shooting fish from trees overhanging the lake water, the hunting of wild turkeys, Junius' unbelievable ability to imitate birds and especially quail until they would come almost within arm's length, dead sure that Junius was one of them, our building of a home-made merry-go-round, his teaching me how to tread water, how to set a dog's broken leg bone, and how to cast bullets.

When I finished, I was sure that I had pushed Junius into his past, and that for the hour we could take up where we had left off years before. I discovered that I didn't know Junius. With a patient gesture, he waved aside my gay items of boyhood. His response was, "As I was saying about pellagra"—and on and on, all scientifically.

"Junius," I said, "so many hundreds of people are aware of your extraordinary medical activities here in this remote country. These people are your great admirers. They love you. There are people who want to come and see you. There are people who would like to take you back to the great centers of medicine to tell of these remarkable things."

Junius was pleased but smiled deprecatingly, "I have been so busy working that I never have time to stop. If anything good has been done, I don't know it."

I gave up the fight to get a glimpse of the old Junius. I was routed, defeated by this dignitary in rags. I left with Junius still safeguarding his ego, remarking: "This summer I think I shall go east, to see some of my friends at Johns Hopkins and later in Boston."

It is highly improbable that at that moment Junius had a penny in his pocket.

I looked about for "the man" needed to guide us through the brush back to the highway. The man had profited the three hours of our visit by emulating the unsaintly half of Junius—he was dead drunk, propped up against the bumper of the car. Such things seem to be endemic in that country.

Alcoholism is no occupational disease of physicians nor any professional group. Thus it slips away from my shrievalty. But, for it, one good word—perhaps it is admirable if it metamorphosed a supernumerary in New York into a highly useful, saintly toper in Alabama—splendid.

Chapter 26

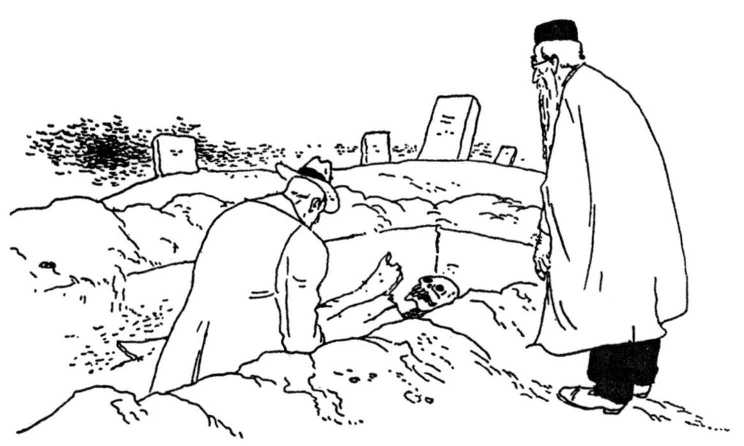

The Doctor and the Rabbi

NOT UNTIL long after the death of some workman may the idea germinate in the minds of his family that the cause of death was related to his work. Often it is too late to derive any conclusive medical evidence through the usual channels of procurement. This may involve the industrial hygienist in the disagreeable process of an exhumation and an autopsy under distressing circumstances. This was the case long after the death of a printer—an orthodox Jew.

Many months after the burial, this dead printer's dependents made legal claims that his death was caused by lead poisoning. Since in life no lead poisoning was known to have existed, nor any clear-cut exposure to lead, this claim appealed to the insurance carrier as unwarranted and was contested. I was consulted and reported that the only reasonable possibility of establishing facts as to lead poisoning was exhumation, followed by a careful chemical analysis of portions of long bones for the detection of stored lead. Even this procedure was so fraught with technical difficulties as to provide many uncertainties.

With the scantiest of knowledge, may I speak with regard to the practices of orthodox Jews in connection with burials. It has been stated, and in this instance seems to be true, that embalming is avoided, that as a last burial action the casket is broken up in order that truly the body may return to the soil from which it originated and that every portion of the body must be interred. It is said to be traditional practice among some persons of this faith to preserve all finger and toe-nail parings during a lifetime in order that these body remnants may be interred after death. Whatever the facts may be, this exhumation was, for the industrial hygienist, attended by unprecedented difficulties.

After necessary legal arrangements had been made, the plan was to exhume the body, bring it into the cemetery chapel, where I was to make such examinations as were possible. It was perhaps unknown to the family that it would be necessary for me to remove from the body portions of bones for lengthy chemical analyses over a period of weeks. The family had arranged for the rabbi to stand guard over the body to make sure that I carried out no desecration offensive to members of that religious sect. However, with an eye more toward money than orthodoxy, the family on the day previous had whispered to me that I should do whatever was necessary and not pay too much attention to the rabbi. Thus this examination was to become a contest between laboratory science and a faithful rabbi.

After hours of digging while the rabbi and I waited in the chapel, the grave diggers in despair reported that it was quite impossible to withdraw the body from the grave. Water had covered the body to a depth of two feet and required frequent bailing. The coffin and outer casing were in splinters. Decomposition left little prospect that the body might be removed except in pieces. We seemed at our row's end.

Quite willing to be of any service possible, I agreed to carry out an autopsy, such as could be done, by entering the grave itself. Donning rubber boots, I descended into the grave and with clean water flushed the mud to some extent from the badly decomposed body. The large quantity of hydrogen sulfide gas from fleshy decomposition threatened to overcome me so that at any moment I expected to fall face forward into the putrifying mess. My autopsy instruments were laid out on a plank spanning the grave. Never have I carried out an autopsy under more disturbing conditions. The set-jawed rabbi watched every movement, rigidly determined that I should not remove any portion of the body.

Despite decay, it was possible to determine that the immediate cause of death had been pneumonia. Both lungs presented characteristic features, leaving no uncertainty in my mind.

While this positive evidence to reasonable minds should have ruled out any further contentions as to lead poisoning, I realized that claims of plaintiffs' attorneys are not always reasonable, and that the plea would be made that both lead poisoning and pneumonia might have existed.

There remained for me the duty of procuring specimens of ribs or shin bones for laboratory purposes. I kept waiting for the rabbi to give up his vigil. The weather was cold, and I anticipated a moment when he might wish to return to the chapel for a respite of warmth. He was faithful to his trust. Not once did he take his eye off my movements. My game was to play for time, hoping for some fortuitous event. For over an hour I did unnecessary things, examination of portions of the body in which I had no professional interest, insisting on more bailing of accumulating water, unnecessary sponging and cleansing of parts.

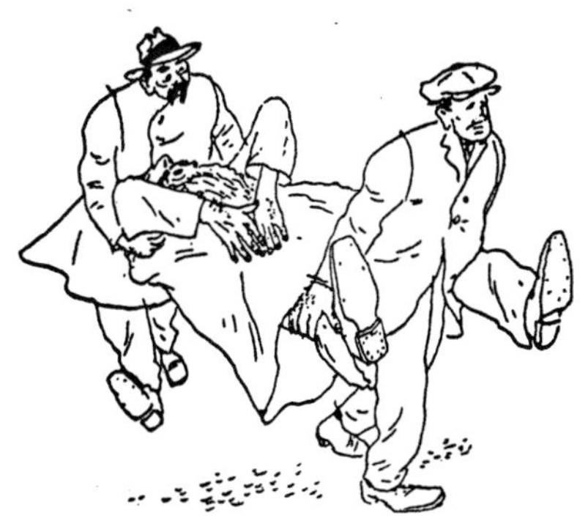

I outlasted the rabbi. Without warning, he fainted, almost falling into the grave with me. Hurriedly he was carried by the two grave diggers into the chapel. This was my opportunity. Quickly I cut away the flesh from two or three ribs and portions of both shin bones. These I thrust inside my boots, completely out of sight. In a few minutes the rabbi, pale, wan, and wobbly, with apparent utter loathing for his necessary task, returned to his post above me. Then I announced the completion of my examination. As I stood beside him, I raised my empty hands, then held before him my tray of instruments. He was convinced that the entire body had been left, if not in repose, at least in its entirety.

Without any sense of guilt, and two-thirds overcome by deadly hydrogen sulfide, I reeled back to the chapel, gloating over the fact that necessary samples of bones were rubbing my ankles, secure in the belief that the rabbi was wholly satisfied that no violations had taken place.

Despite my efforts to conceal identities, it is possible that the good rabbi at this late day may come to know of the advantages that I took of him. If so, I say: "Brother, I apologize. You glued your hawkish eyes on me as long as you were able. I tried to make you faint long before you did. I toppled over two or three times in that grave myself, but you never knew it. Now may we call it square?"

Days later, the chemist came in with a report that no more lead was present than would be expected in the average, unexposed adult. That finding, formally presented to the court, brought to an end the desecration of the printer's last resting place.

Chapter 27

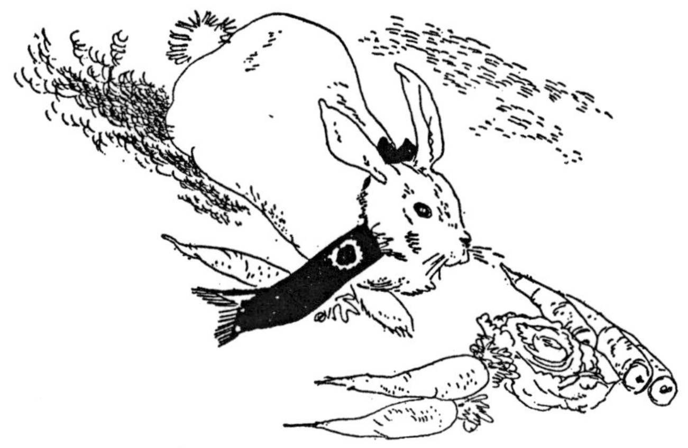

Hammer Head

THE WISEST creature in all the laboratory is Hammer Head. Hammer Head, the senile, arthritic, scraggly rabbit who lives in cage 87, middle tier, north end. Hammer Head, dean of the laboratory animals and sire of the majority. Hammer Head, veteran of endless tests and sole survivor of a two-year animal investigation of wicked industrial gases. Hammer Head, pensioner extraordinary, retired after valiant services to man, amply endowed for the balance of his life with full assurance of plentiful carrots, green food, grains, and vitamins. Hammer Head, dumb contributor to the perpetuation of health for industrial workers.

Such is his citation. Soon I shall propose for Hammer Head, a decoration for distinguished laboratory services. Before this proposal, it is proper to praise the life-promoting contributions of thousands of other laboratory animals in the protection of the more valuable bodies and productive capacities of the industrial worker army.

Whenever I encounter the addle-pated statements of agitators against the use of animals in the safeguarding of human life, I recall the loyalty and faithfulness of one lot of dogs in another laboratory who for weeks had been subjected to various painful procedures in the study of the properties of a little-known substance. These animals were housed in a small building apart from the laboratory. On a day when the cage door, along with the building door, accidently was left open and these dogs were free to escape, to run away from the supposed horror and agony of the laboratory, they did nothing of the sort. In utter faithfulness they rushed to the laboratory building, up the stairway three flights and one by one leaped onto the operating table and lay down for further services.

Devoutly do I regret that a motion picture might not have been made of this unrehearsed show of fealty. It might confound the rabidness of some of the zealous anti-vivisectionists unfamiliar with the hearts of laboratory workers.

Knowing that you will be willing as I am willing to praise my rabbits, guinea pigs, and rats, I ask in their behalf, opportunity to present just one example of their services—the exploration of the dangerous properties of metallic magnesium.

For one hundred ten years after its discovery in 1830, metallic magnesium was contented with lethargy. In 1917 and 1918 magnesium was given a few awakening shakes, but only from the thunders of World War II did metallic magnesium arise to become the magic material for war-winning.

Chiefly magnesium is a gift from Neptune. His resources are unlimited. From eight hundred tons of sea water one ton of metallic magnesium may be derived. This means that if you well filled your big bathtub with sea water you might bathe in a few ounces of dissolved magnesium. From a cubic mile of sea water the number of tons of magnesium obtainable is fabulous — nine billion pounds. The figure frightens me, but you have read the manufacturers' advertisements just as I have.

Magnesium is one-third lighter than aluminum. Thus, it might be possible for one workman to lift a magnesium-built grand piano off the moving van, for a mother to lift a magnesium baby carriage, baby and all, up the apartment steps. Conceivably two men might carry a magnesium-built automobile up onto the front porch out of the rain.

All that is for a future day.

At this writing magnesium has its war history. Alloyed with aluminum and other metals it made the shell of many types of military aircraft, notably bombers.

So suddenly did magnesium spring into full-bloom use that industrial hygienists such as I were caught napping. Vague rumors drifted through roundabout channels of queer happenings in Germany and Italy from the manipulation of metallic magnesium, stories that were hard to believe. Knowing that tens of thousands of war workers in this country would be exposed to pure magnesium and magnesium alloys, it was necessary to determine how dangerous magnesium might be. What harm might befall workers? Would it act like mercury or arsenic or manganese? Not knowing, we politely asked the rabbits and the rats.

Accordingly, some metallic magnesium was ground to fine particle size, so fine in fact that the particles would pass through a hypodermic needle, when admixed with saline solution. In so fine a form, magnesium will oxidize to blackness with readiness, so it was necessary to grind this material and later heat-sterilize it in an atmosphere of nitrogen.

When this material, in small amounts equivalent to the size of a match head, was introduced under the skin, a remarkable thing happened. In a single night rats developed queer gaseous tumors the size of pigeon eggs. This was a thing unheard of, except that this was the rumor that had oozed out of Germany—gas tumors, vacuoles. It was easy enough to withdraw some gas in vacuum tubes from these tumors, and to make suitable analyses. When this was done there were good reasons to believe that the gas within these pockets at the outset was hydrogen, hydrogen liberated from the fluids of the body, the fluids that bathe every cell of the rat's body and yours.

When these tumors were examined microscopically, they proved not to be simple gas pockets but pockets with walls thoroughly necrotic, destroyed by some chemical procedure. Gangrene is the usual name for such a state.

Then it was that the rats and the rabbits were asked to tell why so much extraordinary tissue destruction from the gas tumors. Under anesthesia tiny thermometers were implanted beneath the animals' skin. Around the mercury bulb of the thermometer the magnesium was deposited. The bright concept was that if the heat of chemical reaction was sufficient to cook the tissues to necrosis this would be recorded on the thermometers. Nothing happened. However, in the process the animals did tell the story of why so much damage. In the liberation of hydrogen from water, enough alkali is produced to bring about the damage. Better to prove this, tanks of ordinary hydrogen (not nascent hydrogen), oxygen and nitrogen were procured and, with hypodermic needles properly connected with rubber tubing to the tanks, the same size tumors were produced, avoiding all chemical reaction from metals beneath the skin. But here no gangrene took place, simply mechanical bubbles.

Already much was known, but it was necessary to learn what might happen if magnesium powder by ill luck was ground into the outside skin either in an abrasion of its own making or from some other cause.

Here it was that the rabbits did prime service, since the gas tumor burden in major part had been carried by rats. So, small areas about two inches square were shaved over the rabbits' bellies and these areas were made a little raw, and into this rawness were rubbed the fine magnesium particles. It must have hurt considerably—my own did, but rabbits are stout-hearted soldiers. Into other rabbits were rubbed such other materials as aluminum, zinc, and iron.

In the next day and the next the rabbits began to tell their stories.

Through some peculiar property the magnesium dissolved skin so that the wounds were wet and drippy, but not so the aluminum, the iron, and the zinc wounds.

The rabbits had given us another fact, the fact that magnesium dust is considerably more dangerous than ordinary dusts, and that every effort should be made to avoid wounds from this metal.

More weeks passed, and more rabbits and more rats shouted their evidence of the dangers of magnesium. When enough had been done, all of the little pieces of evidence were put together until no portion of the mosaic was lacking.

Then it was possible to say to all physicians, and particularly those responsible for magnesium workers, "Do not permit splinters of magnesium metal to lie embedded in the flesh. Remove all, even though it be necessary to excise much flesh. If this is not done, gas pockets will be produced, and these gas pockets are slow of healing and will do workers harm, and will slow down the nation's aggressive efforts. And more, do not allow magnesium to be ground into the skin. It will liquefy the skin. The dissolved skin will be slow to heal and the injury will be out of proportion to its apparent severity."

This is the story that the rabbits and the rats told us, and this is the story handed on in the interests of man protection and woman protection. This is one contribution of rats and rabbits to a nation which rightly thinks mostly of people, but wherein even laboratory animals play their role of helpfulness.

Now Hammer Head stands by, looking modestly important. Ray, the deiner, has smoothed his aging furry coat and cleaned out his cankering ears. He nudges Ray's hand, asking that his head be scratched just a little as assurance that all is well. He kicks up his hind legs playfully, trying to convey the impression that he is as good a buck as at the age of eight months, but awkwardly abandons the process as his arthritis grips him.

I ask that you bestow on this paradigm of all good laboratory animals, your highest decoration for meritorious laboratory services.

Chapter 28

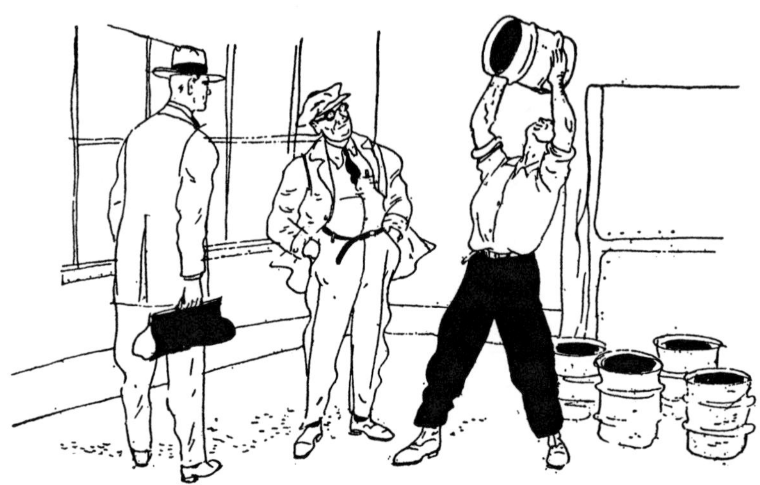

A Minor Medical Miracle

At the Forsyth Storage Battery Company's plant, it was my duty, in return for the small monthly salary paid me, to make examinations of all workers exposed to lead, as required by law in that state. In addition to the routine examination of gum lines, hand grips, weight, skin color, I carried out a basophilic aggregation blood test on a drop of blood carefully spread over a microscopic slide. As to two or three workers I was suspicious that a trivial degree of lead poisoning existed and ordered that their work be changed for the time being to eliminate further exposure. Then I came to Marshall Grant.

From the physical examination, nothing suggested any lead involvement, but up stepped the laboratory assistant who was making the blood examinations. Speaking with much more delight over positive findings than should have been reflected in his attitude toward a possibly sickly man, he said. "Here's one for you, Doctor. Here's a B.A. of seven per cent."

This was important, since in this test, any percentage over one and a half or two suggests the presence of lead.

To Marshall, and to the foreman standing near him, I said, "You look all right, and you say you feel all right, but if this laboratory test is worth anything you ought to be in the hospital."

"Go on, Doc. I never felt better in my life. Watch me." He picked up a fifty-pound tin of lead oxide and raised it above his head.

"Don't bother about me. I'll be all right."

That was Friday morning. On Saturday morning, a phone call came in from the foreman's home, since the plant was not operating.

"You were right about that man Marshall Grant. He's gone crazy. He nearly fell off of a roof. His father just called me from his home down in Kentucky. Maybe he hasn't got lead poisoning. I never heard of anybody going crazy from lead, but you said yesterday that by rights he ought to have lead poisoning, and if he has we ought to know it. Will you drive down those twenty-three miles and find out what it is?"

I would.

I was accompanied on this trip by a young physician, now famous as an investigator of lead poisoning, who then was just starting on a brilliant career.

Far to the south of Erlanger we found this patient in his father's home suffering from manifest and unusually severe lead encephalitis, lead poisoning of the brain which is associated with swelling of the brain within its bony cavity. Three neighbors were attempting to hold him on the bed in

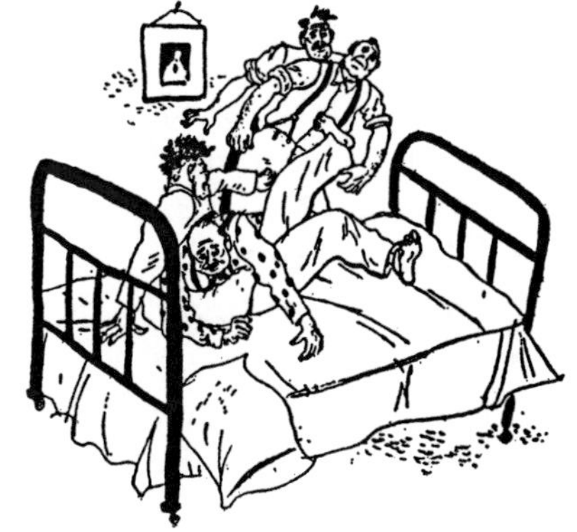

his mania, but being more powerful than all, he was tossing them about with freedom. In complete delirium, he was unable to furnish us any history or description of his condition. To make any examination other than observation was out of the question. As one hand-wringing woman in the sick room remarked, "It takes three persons even to look at Marshall."

The accompanying doctor stated, "I have along some Fischer's solution. If we could just introduce this intravenously, we might be able to reduce brain edema and this man might get some relief, but we could never hope to get a needle in a vein, much less to keep it there long enough to carry out any slow administration of this saline."

From the boy's father we learned that early on that Saturday morning the son, without any illness, had agreed to help in the roofing of the house. Near noon, with no warning, he had gone into a convulsion and rolled down the roof, but fortunately at the point where a heavy ladder lay against the roof edge. There he was caught.

In desperation, the father then threw his own weight against the ladder by standing on it on the outer side from the boy. Calls for help brought two other men working on the farm, with whose aid the boy was lowered to the ground, and thence to bed.

If this had occurred on a summer's day, sunstroke might have been the diagnosis, but cool weather eliminated this diagnosis as a probability. Besides, we were able to take the patient's temperature, but not by mouth, and there was missing the telltale temperature elevation so characteristic of sunstroke.

To the family we expressed the belief that, in this severe mania, death almost inevitably would take place in view of his location in a remote home far from any hospital and because of our inability to carry out treatment on account of continuous violent convulsions.

The family realized the plight of the patient and had seen our futile efforts to carry out even the simplest of examinations. We walked out into the yard to consider any overlooked possibility in the way of treatment. Soon we agreed on a procedure. If we could not give the healing solution intravenously, perhaps with the aid of several persons holding the patient we might be able to introduce a concentrated lot of fluid through the lower intestinal tract.

This we undertook, but it was much of a struggle. Time after time it was necessary to make a new start. Exhausted ourselves, we kept up the fight until we had introduced some three-fourths of the quantity desired. We had little hope that much would be accomplished, but at least we had done that which every good physician should do; we had made every effort.

By this time, it was well into the night. The patient was no better. Again we told the family, "In conditions of this sort, the patient usually dies, and we believe this patient may die and soon." Then we left.

Next day our interest in an unusual case, plus interest in a distraught family and still further consideration for an employer who undoubtedly would be charged with the ignominy and expenses of an occupational disease death, again carried us down into Kentucky. Without pleasure, and with that customary distress that attends any physician when a patient in his charge dies, we came to the house and guardedly asked, "What about Marshall?"

His father, with a great glow of appreciation for us, said, "Oh, Marshall. He's all right, I guess. He's at church now. He got up this morning and said he was all right — he looked all right. That certainly was fine medicine you doctors gave him last night. We thought we were going to lose our boy. He's going back to work tomorrow morning."

We were so unbelieving that we looked in the bed. We waited for Marshall. In truth he was free from all signs of his mania. He was wholly unaware who the physicians were who cared for him the night before.

"They tell me I was pretty 'ornery' yesterday afternoon and last night and caused a lot of trouble. I guess maybe it was something in the shingles."

"No, Marshall," I replied, "do you remember on Friday I told you that I had every reason to believe that lead poisoning was just ahead of you? You talked me out of it. That got us both into trouble. Look what happened to you. The worst is over, but you aren't going back to work tomorrow. You're going to stay right here at home for two weeks at least and we're going to watch you. But remember, don't get up on any roofs."

The hope is that a myriad of people will ask, "What is a B.A. test?" For those thus inquiring, here's what it is about and how it all started.

Chapter 29

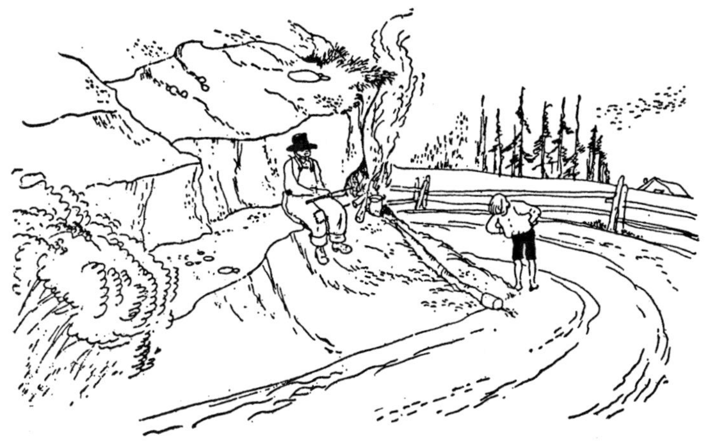

The Birth of the B. A.

ACCIDENT has played so large a part in the discoveries of medicine and science that any elaborately planned investigation is from the outset cursed with the threat of barrenness. Whether the result of accident or of deliberate planning, every scientific discovery has a human and dramatic story that seldom reaches print. Wrapped up in the ponderous garb of dignity, scientific publications seldom reveal the real basis of the discovery.

Around any discovery a score of legends may be built. Every intimate feels that his version is the only true account of what really took place. In time, these legends are transferred to other investigators and other discoveries. Science has its apocrypha, no less than the Bible. In recounting a few instances of discoveries by accident, freely it is ceded that my versions may be apocryphal.

In 1895, Wilhelm Roentgen, of Wurzberg, walked into his laboratory and unconcernedly placed a bunch of keys on top of a group of sensitive photographic plates carefully protected against light. The scientist then went about his chore of the investigation of Crooke's tubes. Later, he exposed those photographic plates. After development, to his disgust, he found that his plates were worthless for the purpose intended, because the image of his keys was on the negatives. Something remarkable had happened. Some unknown ray that must have been present in his laboratory had forced its way through the protective covering of the plates and cast the image of the keys through which the rays did not pass upon the plates. Thus the x-ray was born — through sheer accident, but an accident turned to good account the world over by an intelligent mind.

Until 1889, it was not known that the pancreas was the body organ foremostly involved in diabetes. In that year, Von Mering and Minkowski removed the pancreas from numerous dogs. All were doomed to die, but no one then realized the physiologic processes that necessarily associated the extirpation of this gland with death after a few days. One morning a disgruntled deiner came from the animal quarters to the chief's office and announced he was quitting. Pressed for a reason for his leaving after many years of service, he stated, "I've cleaned up after dogs for years, but when they begin to urinate syrup, I'm through."

The janitor was right. There was syrup in the urine — sugar — the sugar of diabetes. A host of diabetics, now comfortable and without disability in part owe their life to this janitor, disgusted with dog urine with a high sugar content.

Look in any chemical dictionary, encyclopedia or biographic compendium. There will be found the name of Sir William Perkin. Not always was he Sir William, not always was he famous. At Easter time of 1856, the youthful Perkin was at home in England on vacation from his chemical tasks in Germany. With the energy of youth, he had set up in his own home a temporary laboratory. Having imagination, he conceived the possibility of synthesizing quinine, then a much-needed and costly drug in his country — from common coal tar. To various fractions of distilled coal tar, he added divers other chemicals and watched expectantly for results. He did not produce quinine. Instead, there settled to the bottom of one of his beakers a world-changing purple sediment — the first synthetic dye — mauve.

Later, in the world of synthetic chemistry, the greatly desired achievement was artificial indigo. One chemist diligently working from 1865 to 1880 finally created the transformation of toluol (a benzene-like substance derived from coal tar) after many chemical manipulations into synthetic indigo. Important as was this triumph, it was of no direct practical value, for the cost exceeded that of natural indigo.

Another chemist and his assistants took up the burden. They concluded that if the world supply of toluol was insufficient, for a low price starting point and synthetic manipulation a cheaper and more plentiful substitute must be found. The answer was found in "naphthalene" — the material of moth balls. After years of prodigious effort, it was possible to produce within his retorts a substance closely resembling indigo, but still not quite indigo. The last step was the most difficult of all. Thousands of experiments were conducted, seeking the magic that would transform the near indigo into indigo.

One day this chemist went to his lunch leaving the precious substance in charge of a helper, with instructions to stir and take temperatures every little while. In due time the chemist returned — before his eyes was the indigo in pure form. In his absence, the magic had worked. The chemist was frantic — the great problem had solved itself — and he didn't know how. He called his assistant, who had done nothing more than stir and take temperatures. Most perplexing. The chemist read weather charts — looked for open bottles of chemicals in the room — thought of impurities in the glass of his containers — to no avail. The completely made indigo was more tantalizing than the unfinished product.

Finally, the helper, thinking that he had ruined his master's product, confessed that while taking the temperature he had broken the thermometer. Expecting condemnation, he was violently embraced by the chemist — the miracle was explained. Mercury was the magic — mercury was the catalyst that transformed moth balls into indigo!

In all of science, accident seems to be the great investigator.

NOT in this category of great discoveries, but in this category of accidental findings, falls the beginning of the basophilic aggregation test. Near as the nearest microscope, any physician or laboratory technician has available a simple procedure that may contribute to the diagnosis of lead poisoning or lead absorption in any suspected patient. There are those in the field of industrial medicine and hygiene who have labeled the B.A. test (basophilic aggregation test) as not being worth the paper on which its descriptions have been published. There are hundreds of other physicians who find in the B.A. test a faithful servant, aiding in the diagnosis of lead absorption and lead poisoning. Good or bad, right or wrong, the much used and much disputed B.A. test was born by accident.

Ordinarily, inability to read and translate German is a forthright disgrace to any scientist. In my case, this disgrace led to the B.A. test, all because I mistranslated a German publication with the title I still am unable to translate, "Anleitung zur Diagnose in dicken Tropfen."

Missing the entire point in a described technique, I created a new and possibly better method of my own.

Having abundant numbers of frank lead poisoning cases, I applied over and over the German's technique as I interpreted it, looking for a peculiar kind of red blood corpuscle. None was present. Over and over I found a wholly different form of red cell unlike that sought, and of a form and shape wholly unknown to me.

In the midst of scores of tests, I did discover that only small numbers of these unknown blood forms were found in normal blood, but in the blood from lead patients, hundreds were in evidence on every slide. By this time, we were more concerned in our own artifically produced cell forms. Applying the term, for working purposes, of "basophilic aggregations" to these puzzling microscopic objects, I set about the business of determining their relationship to lead absorption and lead poisoning.

All other work was stopped. Hundreds of blood smears were made on young and old persons, men and women, patients sick from all manner of disease except lead poisoning. All of these samples carefully were stained and the basophilic aggregations counted. In the normal, healthy person, always a few were detectable, but only a few.

This completed, I set about the examination of all lead poisoning patients who might be found. To my delight, every acute case of lead poisoning revealed three and five and ten times as many of our basophilic aggregations.

Then it was that I went to many factories where lead was made or used — to white lead factories, red lead factories, paint mills, storage battery plants, potteries. Every worker with any semblance of exposure to lead dust or lead fume was examined.

Then came the great disappointment. Among these workers were some who apparently were hale, hearty, and scornful of any thought of having lead poisoning and yet their blood showed high numbers of basophilic aggregations. The whole matter seemed a failure.

I gave up the test, put away the microscopes, started new enterprises. Disappointed.

Mired in discouragement over the loss of a promising scientific enterprise, I gropingly grasped the concept that our peculiar cells might not only occur among patients obviously sick with lead poisoning, but in those workers who were absorbing lead but still were apparently well. This would mean that for every person who was destined later to have lead poisoning, there was a stage or a time when his approaching disease might be prophesied, possibly avoided. Here was opportunity for prophetic medicine, the detection of a disease that might not bring about the pain of disability until next week or next month. If this were true, the worth of our diagnostic test immeasurably would be increased. A new magic possibly might be introduced into the diagnosis of this one disease — its diagnosis before it appeared.

Back to the lead-using plants, back for more blood specimens, back to the laboratory for more cell counting.

In one plant, an especially rugged and husky worker was engaged in the filling of barrels with powdered white lead. The dustiness of lead about him was enormous. In the examination of his blood, I was able to see as many basophilic aggregations as ever had been seen in any actual case of lead poisoning. I argued, "If this new test is of any value, it is showing that here is a workman grossly exposed to lead dust, who is just about to become stricken."

Then it was I made a daring prediction. To this robust man in the presence of the plant's resident physician, I made the simple statement, "If this test is worth anything you ought to come down with lead poisoning any day now, and certainly within two weeks." The miracle happened — he did.

From that hour on, I have known that there was a field of use for the B.A. test.

A little later, in another plant, where no lead was utilized, physical examinations were being carried out on a group of one hundred and eighty applicants. I still was looking for opportunities to collect samples of blood for control purposes, seeking to establish the normal numbers or percentages of our peculiar cells such as might be found in healthy people. Later, in the laboratory, only one specimen out of these one hundred and eighty samples yielded high numbers of basophilic aggregations. In this one test, there were nine times as many of these cells as found in any other. This applicant's record indicated no possibility of exposure to lead. Rightly discouraging.

Four days afterward, a telephone call came from the plant physicians where the one hundred and eighty applicants had been examined.

"You remember," he said, "the big fellow on whom you found

thirteen per cent of your basophilic aggregations? You said he spoiled your test. He didn't — he's in the hospital now with lead poisoning."

Over at the hospital, the patient, writhing in the agony of lead colic, freely admitted that he had lied in giving his earlier statement that he had been a truck driver. Instead, he had been working with his father and uncle in a petty battery enterprise carried out in the basement of his uncle's home.

Twenty years have elapsed since the first uncertain days with the B.A. test. More than two hundred thousand tests have been made by us on humans, monkeys, dogs, rabbits, guinea pigs, rats, and birds. No test is infallible and this includes the B.A. test. A half dozen diseases other than lead poisoning yield positive results. Newborn babies run high tests until about ten days of age. Over the land, there are more than twelve thousand workers exposed to lead to whom this test has been applied.

The results obtained probably have saved many hundreds of workers from the tortures of lead poisoning. While few patients have been taken into the secret of the accidental finding of this test, all might be willing to join me in a certain amount of satisfaction that I never was able to read German.

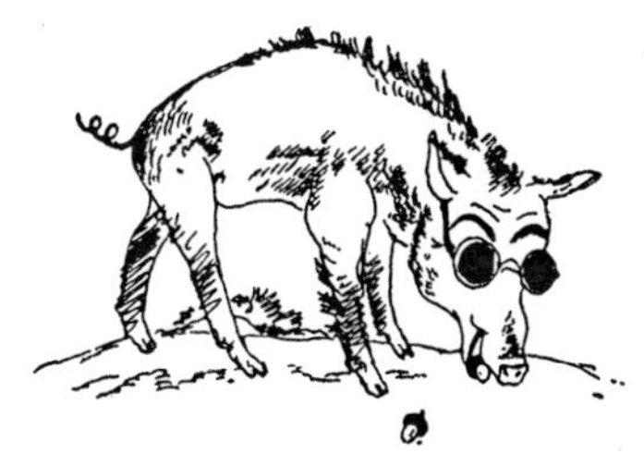

Chapter 30

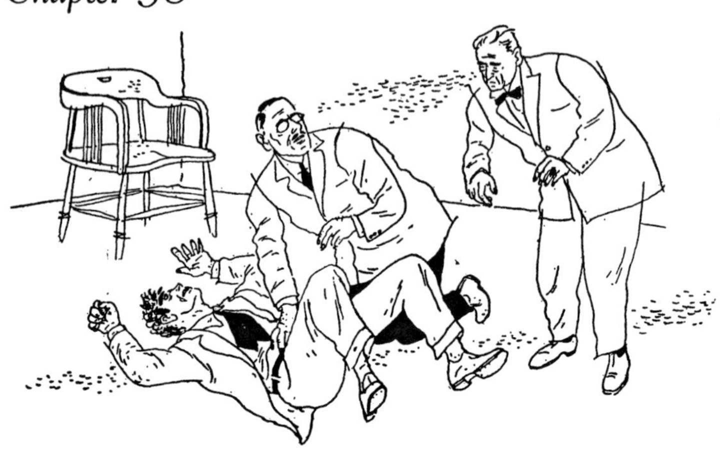

A Reversal in Diagnosis

All included, I probably have had opportunity to participate to some degree in more than 2000 cases of lead poisoning, lead absorption, or alleged lead poisoning. Unquestioned industrial lead poisoning cases seldom get into the courts. Spurious lead poisoning is forever sitting beneath the eye of some judge. In the case of Larry Thomas versus the Crocus Laundry Company, I was a witness for the defense.

Before the trial started, the opposing attorney sought to irritate his opponent or possibly this witness by saying, in our hearing, "I never had a better case in my life — clear-cut, straightforward lead poisoning in every respect. My client is having lead colic right here in court."

Maybe he was, for all we knew, for we had been denied any opportunity to examine him. The defense attorney sarcastically replied, "Let's don't try this case twice. The only time that counts is before the jury, and that hasn't been selected."

In due time, the plaintiff's attorney addressed the jury.

"Ladies and gentlemen," said he, "this case represents a claim at common law, brought by my client Larry Thomas on account of poisoning by lead, lead colic. We will introduce evidence showing that he was a painter at the plant of the Crocus Laundry Company for a period over a year. The plaintiff himself will describe to you his symptoms, and several physicians who have cared for this afflicted man in his troubles will testify as to their findings and will make a diagnosis of lead poisoning. We are asking for the sum of ten thousand dollars because medical testimony will bring out the fact that no lead poisoning victim ever fully recovers, and that as a part of their infirmities they are apt to be sterile and unable to produce children. That fact, in addition to actual disability and loss of time over a period of eight and one-half months is the basis for our claim for this award."

The plaintiff, clearly a sick man or a superb actor, on the stand described his work as an interior painter, using only one kind of paint which was furnished him ready mixed by the plant superintendent. It was his job to paint the walls and ceilings of the company's several plants scattered over the city. The plaintiff testified that he was never called upon to paint machinery, piping, floors or window sashes. All this type of painting was in the hands of other departments. The master mechanic was responsible for machinery painting; the plant fire chief for all painting of piping.

The plaintiff was followed on the stand by his wife, who testified that she had been married three years, but had known her husband for five years prior to her marriage. During that entire period of eight years, she had never known him to be sick until his present illness, that as a truck driver he had an enormous appetite, but soon after he began work as a painter she noticed that he was not eating, that none of the cooking pleased him, that the plaintiff did not sleep well at night, had become irritable and quarrelsome and that she had aborted once just after the time of her husband's first disability.

This wife made a good impression as a witness, particularly in regard to her abortion. This happening is fairly common when the female herself suffers from lead poisoning, and not rare when lead poisoning is limited to the husband.

In time, came a battery of four physicians, three of whom had treated the patient. The last posed as a lead poisoning expert. All testified as to the patient's severe illness, his abnormal cramps, his marked loss of weight, and all made a diagnosis of acute and chronic lead poisoning, attributed to plaintiff's work as a painter. One added, "He is a sick man and should not be here."

During cross examination of the plaintiff, Mr. Sokol, the defense attorney, caused him to state repeatedly that he used one type and one color of paint, furnished in the same type of container, and that he had opened up the containers in all instances. This was important, but he annoyed the plaintiff's counsel until he objected to it as unnecessary repetition and the judge properly sustained the objection.

From the several medical witnesses, defense counsel established the fact that this patient and claimant had never revealed the peculiar purple line at the gum margin which is of some significance in lead poisoning. Nor had anyone gone to the trouble of making quantitative measurement of the lead content of the urine. Blood counts of various sorts had been made, but none was precisely diagnostic of lead poisoning. The various physicians based their diagnoses chiefly upon "lead colic," which they emphasized as being sufficient for them to reach a diagnosis of lead poisoning.

During all of these recitals, the plaintiff from time to time squirmed in his seat, pressed with his hands over his abdomen and occasionally asked for a drink of water. It seemed good showmanship. Being a workman in itself, sometimes, is four-fifths of the law in any claim against a corporation alleging personal injury. Soon the plaintiff rested his case.

At once a witness was called who was the chemist for the manufacturer of the paint. Clearly and simply he testified that, in the paint furnished this laundry company for application to its factory walls, no trace of lead was present as an ingredient. In order to avoid the likelihood of lead poisoning, lithopone had been substituted for white lead. The lithopone, he pointed out, was a mixture of barium sulfate and zinc sulfide. The grey color was obtained through the use of some quantity of carbon black, which contained no lead. The chemist testified that if the color had been yellow, orange, or lemon, some lead would be present in the pigment itself, even though lithopone had been used as the chief solid constituent of the paint.

At a recess for ten minutes, the plaintiff's counsel patted his client on the back and said, "You're doing fine. Let the other side furnish the facts. We'll furnish the testimony."

In the afternoon, I took the stand and was called upon to furnish the results of several analyses of samples of paint taken from various containers selected at random at the chief plant. In addition, results were furnished of the analyses of paint scrapings from the walls of many areas where this painter had applied coatings during his period of employment. In no instance had I found any content of lead beyond the minute trace always present in most minerals, and of a quantity less than one one-hundredth of that quantity regarded as sufficient to induce lead poisoning.

Next I was asked to state the usual and characteristic symptoms of lead poisoning. This I did, pointing out among other items the loss of appetite, the loss of weight, pallor, the lead line of the gums, constipation, weakness, particularly in those groups of muscles used most, such as the muscles of the forearm and usually the right forearm in a right-handed person, headache, severe abdominal pain unlocalized in any one portion of the abdomen, the board-like rigidity of the abdominal wall, peculiar types of blood cells, anemia, excess quantities of lead in the urine and, negatively, the absence of fever, high white cell count and many such other evidences permitting a differential diagnosis between lead poisoning and those conditions that might resemble it.

All the time that I was testifying I was watching the plaintiff, gradually realizing that he was definitely a sick man. It was most unlikely that at a time eight and a half months after any exposure to lead, assuming that exposure may have taken place, he would be suffering from any acute lead colic. His every movement suggested abdominal distress. If he was faking, he was overplaying his case. This certainly was not caused at this late date by any remote lead exposure.

Late in my testimony, Mr. Sokol summed up all of the medical testimony by plaintiff's medical witnesses in a hypothetical question and asked me if from the sum total of the assumptions I was able to make a diagnosis of lead poisoning. Quite sincerely my reply was, "No." Then came the inevitable "Why?" I stated that no exposure to lead had been shown, that the symptoms described by the several physicians were not characteristic of any one disease, but might be associated with many, that many of the characteristic features of lead poisoning had not been mentioned as present, and that in this case proper laboratory tests made at proper times in the course of the disease were requisite.

Then came my cross examination. The plaintiff's counsel realized that my testimony must be broken down. It is not easy to confound a medical witness if he has had considerable experience with the type of affection under court consideration. Always the skilled physician has the advantage of any attorney in any medical situation, not because he is more intelligent, but because the matter in hand is medical. Question after question was directed at me—the validity of analytical methods, atypical types of lead poisoning, the lack of necessity for laboratory examinations in some circumstances. My replies I hope were fair and unbiased.

Finally, the attorney inquired, "Doctor, what other condition besides lead poisoning could have caused this severe, spasmodic pain?"

My reply was, "This patient might be suffering from repeated acute attacks of appendicitis, but I have never had opportunity to examine him."

At that moment, the plaintiff collapsed, fell forward from his chair. He was pallid, sweating. On the floor, in the few seconds before he was removed to a courtroom bench, his knees were drawn up over his abdomen and his hands clenched. Obviously he was in real pain. The courtroom was in confusion, but the judge sensing that this might be a ruse did not immediately adjourn court. Plaintiff's own physician hastily examined his abdomen, pulling up his shirt and undershirt. After a few minutes, being more honest than court wise, and in a voice that he perhaps thought was a whisper, but which in fact reached the judge's ears as well as the jury, this doctor stated to the plaintiff's attorney. "This man has an acute appendix. It may be ruptured. We must get him to a hospital at once."

The attorney addressed the court, "Unfortunately I must ask for a continuation on account of the illness of my client."

That ended the case of Larry Thomas as a claimant for lead poisoning. He did have appendicitis, as proved by an operation, and not lead poisoning.

You may want to label this patient as a scoundrel, his lawyer as a mountebank, his several doctors as perjurers. Nothing of the sort. Quite honestly they all believed that lead poisoning existed. This patient had an abdomen full of genuine pain. It was not his function to know the difference between the pain of lead colic and the pain of appendicitis.

Where then may the onus be laid if any onus exists? Unhappily in the laps of the physicians—not for cupidity, but for failure to obtain the readily available laboratory results that would have ruled out any possibility of lead poisoning. Doctors, like other people, are at times prone to lean on their own opinions and to neglect objectivity.

Chapter 31

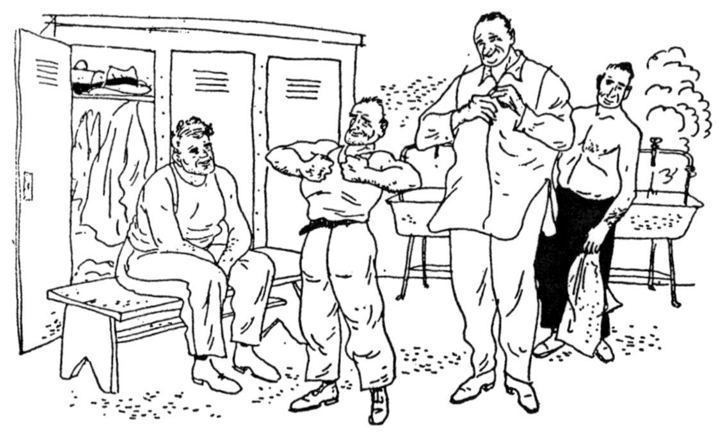

Little Giants

ONE of the sore tragedies that may befall men is to be physically small. In and out of industry these unhappy creatures, loathing themselves and unaware of their "small man complex," spend their lifetimes in fervid efforts to convince the world either that they are not small or, being small, that their prowess excels the six footers.'

Always with exceptions, these five foot giants do strange things that mostly attract attention to their smallness rather than concealing it. No two follow the same pattern, but they are given to moustaches, queer clothes, high-heeled shoes, the cultivation of deep voices, the taking on of physically hard jobs. The big man takes his prowess for granted; the small man daily must demonstrate his. He is an exhibitionist. Look about you on a band. The robust 208 pounder may be happy to play the fife; the 120 pounder may be beating the base drum. Visit a boiler shop. Always there will be one or two distressed souls who subconsciously have elected this heavy work to satisfy their altogether unnecessary shame over smallness. They serve a highly useful special purpose; they can do the inside boiler work.

Nickname, in irony, a strapping six–foot-twoer "Shorty" and his heart will broadcast bruits of delight. Nickname a real shorty "Shorty," and you wrench his heart into agonal silence. If the little man must have an appellation reflecting his physique, call him "Samson" even though he can't lick his height in cellophane.

In industry, the little men, without pre-empting the field of troublemaking for all men and women, provide more than their share. They brashly attempt to show all and sundry that in some magical manner they are beyond the jurisdiction of the factory dangers that threaten ordinary men.

They, more than any other group, are prone to remove the safety guards from buzz saws, childishly believing that such devices draw attention to their childish size. They toss aside goggles, defying any dust particles to affront their superior eyes. They scorn the wearing of respirators provided against the evil action of dangerous duties, gases, and vapors, imprudently challenging the inescapable.

These sixty-two inch Goliaths need no David to throw them. They are highly successful in throwing themselves. As one entry on the ledger of proof, permit this recording.

Up in Marshall County a duck hunter eagerly approached the cabin of his partner who had gone up the evening before in order to have one extra morning's shooting. Both men were from the same factory, the Mason-Corlette Corporation. This was in the days before six-day weeks, when, beginning at four o'clock on Friday afternoon, more than two whole days of recreation might be contemplated.

The second duck hunter found his partner in bed and dead. There were no gun shot wounds. Properly, the unloaded gun stood in the corner. Camp groceries were piled on the kitchen table. There had been a fire in the camp stove, but long since this had burned away.

The police were called, the coroner, the prosecuting attorney, the man's family. The necessary autopsy was performed. Suitable organs were collected and sent to the pathologist of the state university.

Two weeks later this pathologist made his report. Apart from their formal written reports, these pathologists like to be dramatic, and this was a dramatic case. To those assembled in his office, the pathologist stated by way of challenge, "This man was drowned."

Stark amazement appeared on the face of every one there. It couldn't possibly be. There was no suggestion of his having been in water.

"Not the usual sort of drowning, gentlemen," he continued. "This man was not in the water of the lake about his place. No less, he drowned. This man was drowned in the fluid of his own lungs. My examination revealed a gross pulmonary edema. This man was an arc welder. The cause of his pulmonary edema is to be found in the particular work that he performed in the afternoon before he started on his hunting trip. The plant physician where this man worked is present. Let him tell us about this man's work. I have heard the story before, and all details fit perfectly into this picture of tragedy."

Then the plant physician told his story.

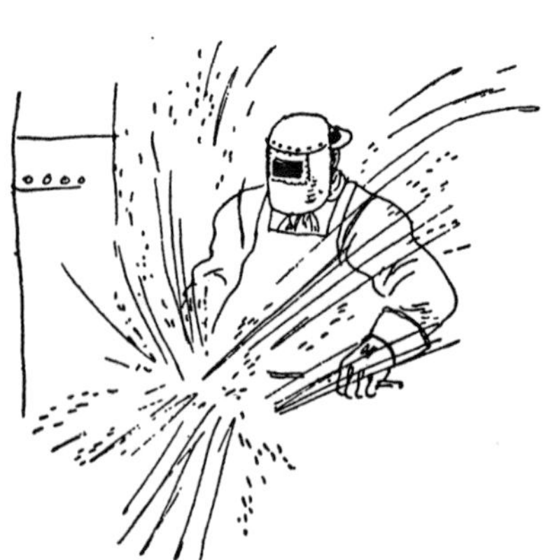

"This man was an arc welder. There are many forms of welding, gas welding with acetylene, spot welding with electricity, thermite welding with chemicals, and others. In arc welding there are many dangers in the absence of well known protective measures. Enough ultra-violet rays are generated readily to produce injuries to the eyes or skin unless the eyes are protected with goggles impervious to ultra-violet rays and unless all exposed skin is covered over with gauntlets, aprons and hoods. All arc welders know this. None goes without this type of protection.

"There are other dangers. Many of the welding rods are coated with dangerous materials. Some of the metals to be welded likewise contain dangerous constituents or are coated with harmful materials, such as fluorides. Most of all, in the arc welding process under the influence of high temperatures and ultra-violet light, nitrogen in the atmosphere is made to combine with oxygen so that abnormal workroom gases are produced, nitrous gases, the oxides of nitrogen. Quantities of these gases commonly are so low so that no harm arises. The threshold of danger is seldom reached. When, however, welding is carried out in confined spaces enough of these gases is built up to bring about disaster.

"We, you know, are ship builders. In ships there are many small cubby holes, compartments, sealed off areas. On this man's last afternoon he was welding but not as usual. He was welding in a small space, only about six by ten feet in dimension. Physically he was a little man. He was given a proper hose mask. He was urged to wear it. He did nothing of the sort. He boasted, 'I've been working for twelve years as a welder and have never been harmed. These fumes might harm some people but they can't harm me. I'm an 'old timer.' These fumes quit trying to get me years ago. I'm too tough.'

"He worked in this compartment irregularly for two hours. Now possibly you want to ask why was not he overcome at once? Why did he not sense his danger? Unfortunately these nitrous gases give no warning of their treachery. They act insidiously. Their harm is delayed. This man left the plant at the regular time at four o'clock. He was excited over his prospective trip. Promised every man in the department one duck. All during the late afternoon he probably was without any discomfort. Somewhere along his route he bought his groceries, enough for himself and his partner for two days. At his cabin he probably went to bed early after having set his alarm clock for five o'clock, getting ready for shooting at sunrise. Before he went to bed he pulled his rowboat out of the boathouse to get water-soaked. He oiled his gun. Everything was being made ready, but what was ahead of him he little guessed.

"Probably by midnight his condition had well started, although that is a guess. If some doctor had gotten to him then, maybe he could have been pulled through.

"He must have died two or three hours before his partner found him at noon."

Then the coroner, who after all was in charge of the inquest, took up the story.

"Just to clinch this diagnosis, we had one other trick up our sleeves. There are some other causes of pulmonary edema, few of which operate quite so rapidly. We had specimens of this dead man's blood on hand for examination. We knew that if nitrous gases had caused this pulmonary edema and this death, we would find in the blood a peculiar substance not normally there, methemoglobin. We found methemoglobin in abundance. The diagnosis is perfect, conclusive."

Diseases, and particulary occupational diseases, leave behind them telltale markings just like other criminals. These pave the way for exact medical diagnoses. Doctors delight in precise diagnosis, but any pleasure is curtailed by distress over the end results of the foolish feats of the arrogant. Their days are numbered.

Chapter 32

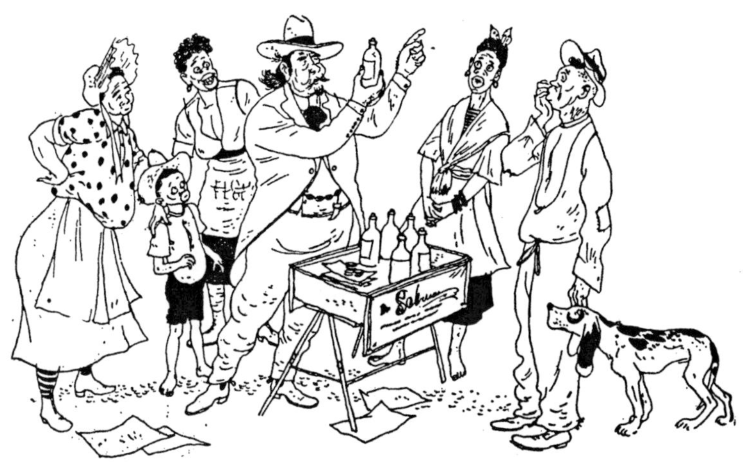

Black Turns White

THE WISE physician always doubts the unusual. The moment the physician begins to feel that he has before him a case of some disease so rare, for example, as leprosy or Kaposi's tumor, professional skepticism should seize him.

This dictum of doubt applies to occupational diseases. Here just a little more leeway is warranted, for almost anything can happen in the way of unheard of diseases.

When I saw my first case of dermatitis from chlorinated naphthalene, I disbelieved what was immediately before my eyes—a workman with outgrowing comedones. In mild degree he was starting a growth of ten thousand tiny horns. In time he might become a human chestnut bur. He did nothing of the sort, but made the beginning.

From such experiences, multiplied a dozen times over, I have learned to hold my receptive antennae in readiness to accept until disproved, some seemingly preposterous industrial diseases. If some foremen were to report to me, "A new chemical in my department is causing two or three of my men to grow teeth in their stomachs like crawfish," I hope my attitude would not lead me to say, "Stupid, ridiculous, forget it," but instead to say, "Let's get an x-ray. Maybe what you say is true."

Without batting an eye I accepted as possible the word brought in by the safety engineer, "In four of our plants in this district, where metal degreasing is done, we have groups of negroes who are apparently turning white."

My reply was, "If that's true, let's get the patent rights. You and I together will make a million dollars a year turning black ones into white ones."

The safety engineer was not impressed any more than I by any real possibilities of monetary gain, but he was impressed by my apparent instantaneous acceptance of his statement.

"No one else to whom I have told this story," he remarked, "will believe a word of it. One or two have said, 'Damned liar,' 'You are seeing through the white of your eye now,' 'How do you get like that?' Then I come to you, Doctor, and apparently you regard the story as plausible."

"At least it's possible," I interrupted, "but let's get at the facts."

Here I was confronted at last with the negro's age-old problem, how to get rid of his stigmatizing color. With emancipation from slavery, somehow or another many negroes believed that they likewise should be emancipated from blackness. Some of the most cruel medical charlatans have been those who, in the decades after the war between the states, preyed upon the yearnings of hopeful negroes by selling to them chemicals guaranteed to turn them white. The lucky ones were those who received for their hard earned money nothing more than a harmless ointment, the humbug having moved on out of reach. The unlucky ones were those furnished a sharply acid lotion or salve which through actual partial destruction of skin produced a spotty whiteness.

In a few sections of the country, two or three decades ago, it was common to see whole groups of piebald or calico negroes. Foolishly seeking to emulate the better faring whites, these negroes wishfully applied these destructive agents to their faces, necks, and hands. The results were pathetic — burning pain, suffering and scarring. The pitiful outcome rather than making whites out of negroes merely served to accentuate the negro skin qualities and to advertise their dissatisfaction with their racial lot.

All this passed through my head as I set about plans for the investigation of this amazing report brought in by the safety engineer.

At the very first of the plants visited, the report proved to be quite valid. Here both negroes and whites were engaged in the cleansing of metal parts in naphtha. Naphtha is an irritant, so that this work calls for the wearing of protective aprons and gauntlets. Naphtha itself could never be the cause of the skin blanching because for years many tens of thousands of workmen daily have gone about duties providing skin contact with naphtha. If this skin whitening could have been produced by naphtha, this would have happened years ago and to many persons.

I asked to see some of the worst cases. In they came. Startlingly striking was the appearance of some because of the sharp contrast between the deep black of normal skin and the utter pinky whiteness of some other portions of the skin. No albino was ever whiter or freer from pigment. It was amazing. There was no soreness, no inflammation, no redness, just whiteness.

Here appeared to be a new occupational disease — chemical leukoderma. But what chemical?

Then came the inevitable questioning, the usual interrogations of the industrial hygienist.

"What is your job? What are you doing that is different? When did this condition first appear?"

With the aid of the foreman, as well as the patients — perhaps we should call them subjects rather than patients, since they were neither sick nor disabled — the story became comparatively simple.

The foreman acted as spokesman, "All the workers in my department have to wear gloves and aprons — sometimes boots. Naphtha softens up ordinary rubber, so that some gloves didn't last two hours. We were costing the company a small fortune just for gloves and aprons. Then we were told they had a new kind of glove that wouldn't be limbered up by naphtha. Everybody liked this new kind — they lasted much longer. But slowly, and we don't know when it began, nearly everybody began to turn white in spots, but only where the rubber touched. The colored boys got white and the white boys got whiter. At first we called them 'liver spots,' but they got too big for that. We didn't pay much attention to it because nobody got sick. Now we believe it is this new kind of rubber that's whitening them out."

This was clear-cut, scientific testimony. Manifestly from the distribution of the depigmentation, the cause was somehow related to the new gloves or aprons. I wanted to know more.

Here was a group of men with white splotches over their hands, forearms, chests and abdomens. I inquired, "What happens when you go out in bright sunshine? Do you get badly sunburned?"

"No," came the reply, "we get whiter."

"Has anybody left this department and gone to work on other jobs? What happens then?"

The foreman took up the discussion.

"Three boys have been transferred to other work for one reason or another. One of them regained his usual color, but two of them are just as white as ever and haven't changed a bit in six months."

While this queer happening was coming to me as a new experience, the same event was occurring in other places, particularly in one tannery. All of this ably has been reported by McNally, and by Schwartz, the dermatologist, and his associates. To them, full credit is due for unraveling the highly technical chemical circumstances that brought about this phenomenon. Their wider experience with negroes, Mexicans and white Americans has furnished exact proof that monobenzyl ether of hydroquinone, used by the manufacturer to prevent oxidation of rubber, is the guilty chemical. In innocence, the manufacturer introduced this chemical needed in the production of a more durable glove, wholly unaware of any special propensity to the destruction of skin pigments.

No two scientific groups ever are likely to reach the same conclusions in any situation. Schwartz and his associates found that soon after the termination of exposure repigmentation happily occurred. I hope that they are right and I'm wrong, but in my dozen of cases only two have recovered normal skin color and ten after more than twelve months' freedom from the use of these gloves have unmatched spotty skins.

Unlike women, how patient and unconcerned male workers are over cosmetic damage from any cause. Among my twelve men, there has not been a whisper of discontent. Some time ago I hunted up one white patient to determine if any new growth of pigment was taking place. He was quite skeptical that there was any connection with the wearing of gloves.

"Doc," he said, "you can't fool me and make me believe that those gloves caused the trouble. These spots are 'liver spots.' My grandma had them long before me. You doctors think you know everything, but you don't. Right here up this line is a man with spots who has had them for twenty years and he never did wear these new gloves. Do you want to see him?"

Of course I did, because this promised the finding of a new case.

"There he is up there — the man with the hunting cap on — go up and talk to him. Maybe you'll get set right on this business."

The man in the hunting cap did have widespread spots of albino-like skin, and indeed by his own story he had had them for twenty years, but his was a different disease — vitiligo, a disturbing affair possessed by many persons far removed from factory work and the day by day wearing of rubber gloves.

A little wistfully an unafflicted negro cautiously inquired, "Doctor, could you make me a white man with this same sort of rubber? Could you melt it out of the rubber and put it all over me, over my face and ears and legs? Then would I be a white man?"

"Stay as you are. Stay as God made you." I strongly urged. No physician has any right to play at being God.

Chapter 33

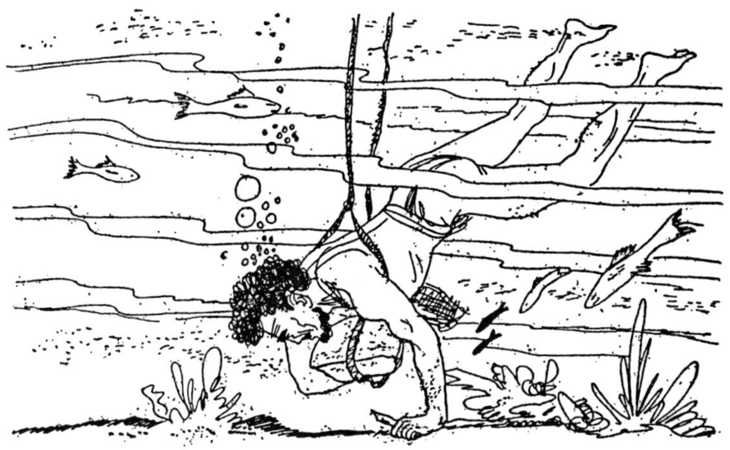

La Maladie de Skevos Zervos

MUCH of medical history is made by little suspecting physicians in the midst of routine duties. Only later does it become history when the matter takes on importance and medical writers delve into origins. The great desideratum is that the physician may possess the mental adroitness that will identify newness as newness, so that a small flag may be hoisted, stele erected, or cairn built and labeled "mine."

With all succeeding crops of medical students it has been my privilege to instruct, always I have plead:

"Go out and find your own new disease. You may remove a thousand tonsils or repair a thousand hernias and still be small fry in the profession, adored by patients, important in the community, prominent in the county medical society — still small fry. Conversely, discover a new disease or a new facet on an old disease, write a few reliable descriptive publications and you become a national character.

"There are plenty of unknown diseases yearning to be discovered — particularly in the realm of occupations. Dr. Towey, living in an upper peninsula town of Michigan, too small to appear in most atlases, traced an obscure lung disease to a fungus growing beneath the bark of saw logs. Today that finding and its finder are known wherever chest diseases are investigated.

"Dr. Sander, of Milwaukee, found among welders unexposed to silica, an x-ray replica of silicosis. This rarely encountered 'siderosis' now known as 'Sander's disease' has removed that young physician from any possibility of obscurity."

For many decades the medical profession made a fetish of attaching the name of the medical discoverer to the discovery. Actually this reflects no immodesty on the physician himself. Instead, his colleagues usually were responsible. Many hundreds of diseases, tests, signs, and symptoms are chiefly known by the discoverers' names. There was a period wherein a physician scarcely might be accorded a place among the mighty unless his name was attached to at least one medical entity. "Basedow's disease" is the common name for exophthalmic goiter. This honor is challenged by some adherents who elect to associate the honor of first description upon Dr. Graves or Dr. Parry. Thus, textbooks variously may refer to Basedow's disease, Graves' disease or Parry's disease. The Italians not to be outdone claim Flajani first described the disease in 1800. At least a dozen physicians' names are associated with different diagnostic signs connected with this one disease. Known to every physician is Graefe's sign, Stellwags' sign, Moebius' sign, Guttman's sign, Jeffery's sign, Hurt's sign, Bryson's sign. Almost any other disease might be presented in terms of names of the physicians who have made contributions, but the dermatologists seem to have been the worst offenders.

Ever there are demurrers. In profound martyrdom they wish to give all to humanity. For them, the reminder that fifty per cent of the capacities of a great man may far overbalance one hundred per cent of the puny minded "wart-hog" variety. Others, with modesty are sure that their small heads will lead them to newness in medicine.

For them, in staunch belief that new occupational diseases may be found almost anywhere, I have the story of Dr. Skevos Zervos, a Greek physician whose far-away contribution finds honor in my appraisal.

For many years the sponge fishermen of the island of Calymnos (in Grecian waters) who search for sponges off the islands of Crete and Chypre and in the African seas, have lived in dread of a strange disease which seemed to attack only sponge fishermen. This disease first manifests itself by a sharp stinging pain at almost any portion of the body, but chiefly on the anterior regions. Quickly this initial spot becomes red and swollen and within a few hours may change in color from red to purple to almost black. Within a short time, systemic involvement arises, characterized by headache, nausea, intense fever and chills, sometimes lasting for several days or weeks. The pain is usually general, is most intense about the open wound, which is slow to heal, prone to necrose, and may eventuate in an abscess. Attacks of this character again and again have been the lot of these sponge fishermen. While death is only occasional, the intensity of the pain is such as to make these fishermen continually apprehensive as they go about their work.

First in 1903 Skevos Zervos presented a description to the Second Panhellenic Congress, and again in Paris at the Academy of Medicine. In the ensuing years, Dr. Zervos has established many unusual features of the nature of this disease and its control. The cause was found to be an animal parasite, the "actinion," belonging to the Zoanthes, and homogenous to the Actinidea. This parasite is approximately four or five centimeters in length. Two rows of minute fingerlike projections occasion the name "actinion," which signifies "ray" formation. This parasite lives attached to the roots of the sponges at the bottom of the sea. As the sponge fisherman uproots the sponges and fills the net bag hung around his neck in front of his body, the disturbed actinion stabs its victim and discharges from its mouth its venomous material, which is described as "white, of viscous consistence, like half-dried nasal secretion." The actuality of poison within the parasite is attest by the use of dried actinions by these fishermen for killing off undesirable animals, such as rabid dogs, etc. Dr. Zervos describes various types of treatment, such as "cupping" the fresh wound, the application of liquid ammonia, etc. It seems somewhat bizarre that with so large a parasite these fishermen should not long ago have determined the cause of this malady. Whatever may have been their extent of knowledge, much has been accomplished by

Dr. Zervos in protecting these fishermen. Through education, through improved therapeutic measures, through prevention of infection, through careful supervision of the sanitation of boats and docks, this disease, never direful, has been brought under control. In gratitude, the population has termed their occupational disease the "malady of Skevos Zervos." The author in turn has dedicated his small book "A mes tres chers compatriotes Calymniotes qui ont subi par milliers cette maladie."

The challenge of interest is a prime quality of any publication. At every turn, this little book extends that challenge. Apparently a remotely situated physician finds an unknown disease; he determined the cause, classified the parasite, established the manifestations, created a suitable treatment, and banished the fears of an apprehensive population. Written in a simple, naive style, it contributes its own small bit to the solution of occupational disease problems.

All this derives from a queer twenty-nine page booklet entitled "La Maladie de Skervos Zervos ou Maladie Des Pecheurs D'Esponges Nus." By the standards of medical ethics and editing in the United States this booklet appears ridiculous — more like a compendium of testimonials for a patent medicine. Governed by the standards of Athens, Greece, the author has seen fit to include in facsimile all his letters of commendation and congratulations. Most of us who write scientific papers never receive letters of commendation, so that this entire paragraph may represent only sheer jealousy.

This is scant praise for a pioneer, a true physician, a servant to the people around him. There are always among us, including physicians withal, those who decry the passing of opportunities for pioneering, new fields to explore, new services to be rendered — the passing of romance in work.

To these pessimists, I would hand a copy of Dr. Skevos Zervos' booklet and say, "The world of opportunity has just begun." Most of all, this booklet from a far land, lends purpose to the present writer's oft repeated contention that occupational diseases may be found anywhere, in all trades, among all classes of workers, and under the most unexpected circumstances.

Chapter 34

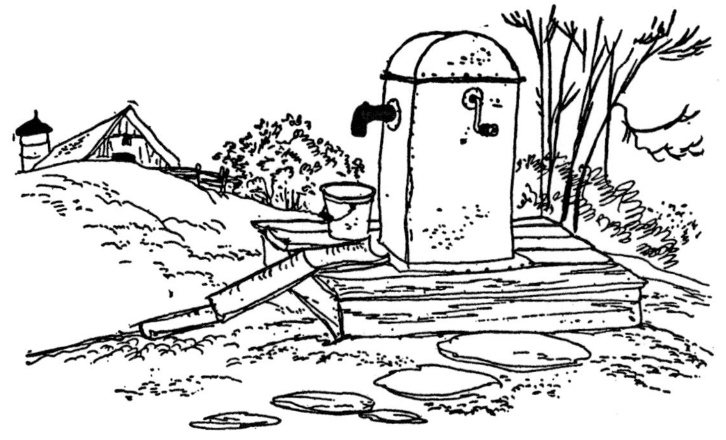

Arsenicism

AT THE hospital, in the "Doctor's Room," which after all is the place where more medical information is swapped than at any academy of medicine, I was awaiting the arrival of my patient with phosphorus poisoning from the fireworks plant.

Since the fourth of July massacres have dampened the ardor of the public for fireworks, except for professionally conducted displays, the fireworks industry, save for military products, has joined the list of dying trades, so perhaps it is not remarkable that neglected conditions led to this case of "phossy jaw."

My patient was late. In came Dr. Wildman, straw hat in hand, which he traded for his long white coat taken from his locker.

"What do you know about shoemakers?" he asked.

"What kind?" I wanted to know. "The one who repairs shoes downtown, chiefly putting on rubber heels, or the one who actually manufactures shoes out at one of the big factories?"

He thought a minute and responded, "The first kind. I've got a man upstairs in the ward who runs a shop in the basement of the Mills Building, who looks like he isn't long for this earth. Anything about his trade that might have poisoned him? I don't know what's wrong with him. I'm willing to have help from anybody. Do you want to see him?"

Upstairs in the male medical ward behind screens, which always are a bad sign unless a patient is having a bath or taking an enema, we found the shoemaker.

Sick as he was, the shoemaker was able to talk and to give good answers to many questions.

But that's getting ahead of the story. First, with proper caution, I asked Dr. Wildman to tell me about his patient. In the manner of the medical professor, which he was, he began his lecture. Gladly I was the student.

"We have here an obviously sick man who has been in the house for ten days. Notice his bronzed skin, which belies that fact that blood counts show that he is somewhat anemic. He has lost a great deal of weight, forty-seven pounds to be exact. Both his arms have lost their motor function, but sensation is well present — in fact this patient's chief complaint is from pain along various nerve trunks which I believe means neuritis. His legs are likewise paralyzed, and when he was brought here he came in an ambulance. If you will notice his nails you will observe that several are missing and there is considerable ulceration around the nail beds. This probably is due to fungus disease. He has lost a lot of hair from his head. I have known this man for years and only a year ago he had twice as much hair as you and I put together. He is about in our class now. At the present time he has a marked diarrhea, which makes it difficult for us to handle him here in the ward. He ought to be in a private room, but he can't afford it. It's hard on the other patients."

Being a little anxious about my own patient, and looking out the window whenever the sound of a newly arrived car was heard, I inquired, "What do you make of it, what is the cause of all this?"

"So far we've been regarding this as pernicious anemia, one of those spinal cord types. The skin isn't quite right, the blood picture is a little off, but not enough to upset that diagnosis. Gastric analysis shows practically no acid, which again suggests P.A. For a while I considered the possibility of pellagra, but this man lives out on a farm which his sons operate, and I know the table they set out there. There couldn't possibly be any deficiency disease here, so that's out. What do you make of it?"

It is always unfair to ask a visiting physician that question. Here I was with only ten minutes' familiarity with the patient's condition against his ten days of intensive study. Besides I realized that Dr. Wildman was chiefly concerned to show me an extraordinary case. No less, I had an idea.

I inquired, "Doctor, do you mind if I ask your patient a few questions?"

"No, go ahead. He's pretty sick, but it won't harm him. Mr. Serpidon, my friend the doctor here wants to talk to you."

Then I began, "Where is your farm?"

"Out the Piper Highway about twelve miles."

"Out in the Moss Hill country?"

"Yes, right among the tallest of the hills."

"How many other members of the family are there besides you?"

"Wife and two grown boys; one of them is married and they have two children, and that's all."

"Do any of them have any disease anything like you have here?"

"They're not sick at all."

"Do you do any of the farming?"

"Hardly a lick. I have to stay in the shop six days a week. Once or twice this year I've driven a haywagon on Sunday, or maybe it was a holiday."

"Besides raising hay, what sort of farming do the boys do?"

"They don't do much farming either. They mostly raise apples. All that country is apple country you know."

"Do you spray your fruit trees?"

"I don't, but the boys do. They spray with some sort of arsenic solution, four or five times a year."

"You didn't help any this year?"

"Not an hour."

"You weren't out there any time that spraying was going on?"

"Maybe as much as an hour or two."

At this point Dr. Wildman broke in. "I thought of arsenic poisoning just as you do and thought of the fruit tree spraying, but Mr. Serpidon here was out there less than anybody else. He was always away except at night. The rest of the family were always present. That seems to rule out any exposure there."

I was a bit baffled myself as to exposure, but I continued, "Mr. Serpidon, are you getting tired? Can you stand a few more questions?"

"Is your house on top of a hill or in flat country? How is your house located?"

"At the foot of a hill with the orchards running up behind the house."

"Let us leave your house alone for a little while and talk about you work. You don't tan any leather in your shop, do you?"

"Not a square inch. Sometimes I dye shoes."

"Those dyes are sometimes harmful, but they wouldn't produce any disease like this. Let's forget about it. What else do you do at your shoe shop?"

"I mostly wait on the customers and the other workers do the actual repairing. I don't touch one pair of shoes a day unless we get in a rush."

That lead seemed to come to a dead end.

"Let's go back to your home. Is there any possibility that any of that arsenic might have gotten mixed up with your food?"

"Not a chance. All the spray machinery and chemicals are kept out in the apple house in the spring. That's all cleared out before harvest time and put in a shed off the barn."

"What sort of water supply do you have?"

"The rest of the family like well water and we have a deep well on the place, four hundred feet deep. Good limestone water for those that like it. I don't like it. I drink cistern water."

"You're the only one that drinks cistern water?"

"Yes sir."

"Any cooking done with cistern water?"

"No, the women folks use it to wash their hair because it's soft but that's about all they do use it for. That cistern was on the place when we bought it, but none of the rest of them can stand cistern water — too flat. We had the well drilled the first year we were there."

"That's all, Mr. Serpidon. Many thanks. Dr. Wildman and I will think this over."

Back in the "Doctor's Room," Dr. Wildman looked up expectantly, "I think I know what you're driving at, but what's going through your head, Doctor?"

"Can't be sure, but it all fits."

"What fits?"

"If this isn't arsenic poisoning, it's a dead ringer for it."

"Where did he get it? Nobody else out there is sick. He goes away and they stay at home. He's sick and they are well."

"Out of the cistern water."

"How would the arsenic get there?"

"The house is at the foot of the hill. This sprayed orchard lies behind the house on the hill — the spray just settled on the roof and the first rain washed it down."

"Good Lord, maybe you're right. What can we do?"

"Have the water analyzed immediately. Also cut off some of his hair, and have that analyzed for arsenic."

An orderly was at the door calling to me. "Your patient is here, Doctor. He's up in 47."

Two days later, Dr. Wildman met me in the hallway.

"You were right. Enough arsenic in that cistern water to kill anybody in time. Even if it wasn't there, we found plenty in his hair. But tell me this, how in the world were you able to figure this out?"

"No credit to me," I replied. "I saw a case just like it in Indiana last summer. Down in 47, I've got a mild case of phosphorus poisoning — come down and have a look."

"Thanks, I will, Doctor, but to even up the score, I ought to prove that your patient has pernicious anemia."

Chapter 35

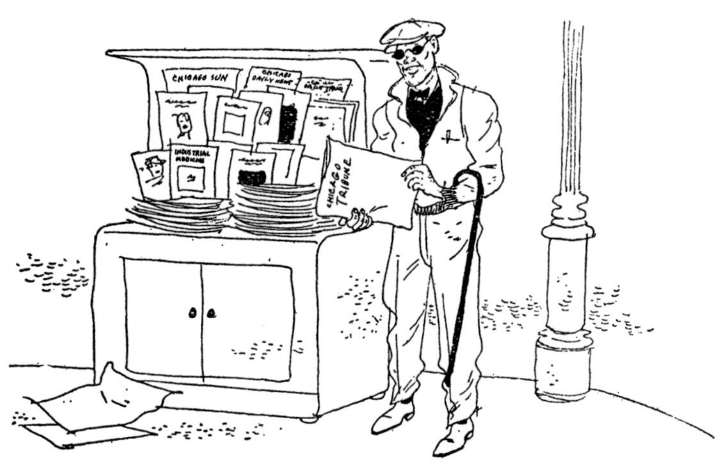

Blindness from Benzol

YES, I know the blind newsman with a stand at the corner. To many he is just "the blind newsman." To me he is more. Once long ago, nearly twenty years now, he was my patient. He was fully blind when I first saw him, which fact removes the curse of any observation that if he had had a better doctor he might not now be blind.

Elmer Broadhead, for that is not his name, is modestly successful, has been paid some thousands of dollars by his former employer, all that the law provided. Elmer is far too busy to tell his story. Besides he is none too anxious to dig up his past. So, I offer myself with some knowledge of his medical history.

"Elmer, before he was twenty, worked at a bakelite plant making laminated bakelite. That was more than twenty years ago. In those days, bakelite was much used in radio cabinets. It was one of the first popular plastics. Bakelite, as you know, is one of these queer man-made resins made out of carbolic acid-phenol-formaldehyde. To make this resin thinner so it could be coated onto sheet fabrics, it was diluted by benzol, along with some other solvents. Benzol is not used any more for this purpose, thank goodness. Other solvents are better and safer.

"This benzol is almost head-man in the troublemakers among solvents. In this same plant where Elmer worked and got into difficulty, three or four deaths occurred in his department.

"Benzol is no friend of the human body. High concentrations of its vapors such as in a tank car may have you down in five minutes, and after ten minutes your entire future may depend upon how you have spent your past. From lower amounts such as you might hardly notice around a workplace, slowly there may come about a chronic disease with a lot of unusual happenings. One of the commonest is that you may bleed under your skin, or into your skin, until you look a little like a human leopard or, more likely, like you had fallen down a long set of icy steps, hitting each step at a different place. Elmer had some of these skin hemorrhage splotches. Other people go in for bleeding from various parts, into the stomach and maybe into the bladder. Women mostly bleed from their genitalia, which is always alarming. If they are pregnant they may abort. Most everyone will bleed from his gums, particularly if he has any bad teeth. That is not all that benzol does, but that is the only body onslaught that we need to talk about in Elmer's case.

"Through some damnable choice on the part of Elmer's body, the place for his benzol hemorrhage was ruinous. A hemorrhage itself is not necessarily serious if it happens to involve the stomach (although any benzol poisoning serious enough to produce a gastric hemorrhage is no inconsequential matter), but when unhappily the hemorrhage is into the back chamber of the eye, and, more unfortunately, both eyes, what can you do? You can't drain an eyeball like an abscess. You can't empty an eyeball like a wen on the scalp. Elmer's hemorrhages were clear-cut and disastrous. Elmer doesn't know this. Month by month he waits for his returning eyesight. If his present physician is the kind-spirited soul that I believe he is, he will share with this blind boy the hope that a miracle may happen, that eyesight may return."

THERE are only a few Elmers from benzol. Those few taught the great lesson that unless harnessed in its proper work sphere, benzol is a felling miasm, striking down all who long accept its malignant presence. Elmer is a disabled veteran in the war to provide work-places free from the prospects of disaster.

Elmer is a little proud of his contribution. "Doctor," he once said, "they tell that out at the plant after what happened to me they rebuilt everything."

They did. I have seen it, but Elmer hasn't. Elmer's blind.

Chapter 36

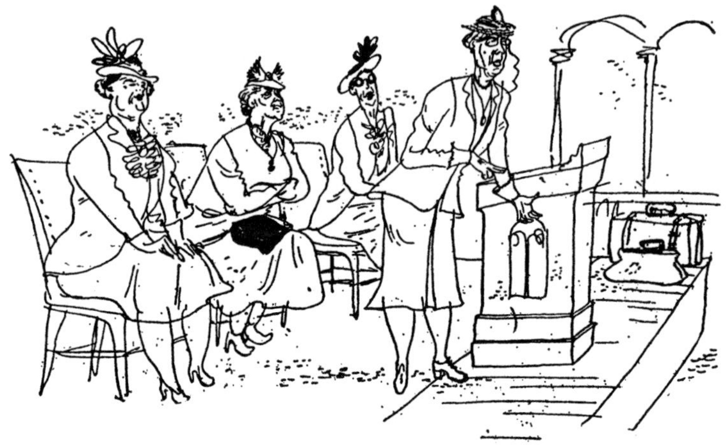

Metal Fever

On the night before this unexpected happening, I had given a talk before the local medical society at Wrexford. The last train toward my home had left Wrexford long before the end of my talk, so that I spent the night at a local hotel. The next morning I had started out on the accommodation train with the prospect of boarding a fast train at Barron eighty miles away, after an hour's wait at that point. At this junction, an enthusiastic group of ladies with some of the earmarks of religious crusaders met a fellow passenger of mine, obviously a prospective speaker for some meeting. After the excitement of ebullient greetings, all the women departed and I looked about for my hand baggage, which I had placed on the railroad platform. It was gone.

Much concerned, I rushed about, inquiring of the station agent. Fortunately, he remembered that the two pieces of luggage I described had been carried off with the luggage of the woman speaker.

With small town prescience, the agent knew that my belongings probably rested in the anteroom of the Calvary Methodist Church. There were no taxis, so I walked eight blocks in the direction given me. When I tiptoed into the church, there was my baggage along with several other pieces, not in any anteroom, but down at the front in plain sight at the right of the rostrum. There was polite nothing to do but wait until the speaker had concluded.

Heatedly, one townswoman, apparently speaking as a preliminary to the visitor, was saying, "Before the coming of the metal works to this town, drunkenness was practically unknown. Our men were a sober lot. Now it is a daily occurrence to see a few drunks after work hours, spending their money on beer and whiskey, neglecting their wives and shaming their children. Their health is being undermined, and it is being rumored that a malaria epidemic has broken out. Nearly all of these drinkers are from a gang of men known to be employed in galvanizing. Apparently this company has specialized in employing these sots, or else it is because they have more money than ever before to buy liquor. Many of us who feel that we are of the better element of the community wish that our formerly quiet village might have been left as it was before the coming of these metal works."

Here was a challenge indeed. This well-meaning speaker could not have realized that there was no malarial epidemic among these workers or that an incentive to alcoholism possibly was being provided these workmen by the work itself.

But these things I knew and after my baggage was rescued by the sexton, who appeared at this time, and to whom I whispered my predicament, I hunted up the manager of the unpopular metal trade factory. Already I had missed my train.

To him I recounted my experience with the ladies at the church. Their unfavorable attitude was not news to him and he was genuinely concerned.

He said, "It is true that the workmen in our small plant do a lot of drinking. There is a great deal of absenteeism among them, and we attribute this to their drinking. Many of them have attacks of some disease that around here is called malaria, but to me this seems unusual, as we are far out of any malarial district and nobody except our workers seems to suffer from the disease."

When I explained that I was an industrial hygienist and somewhat familiar with the unusual diseases that sometimes arise in connection with work, he urged me to stay over and investigate his situation. He invited me to put up at his house, since there was no hotel, and volunteered the payment of adequate compensation for any services.

During the afternoon, I interviewed several of the workmen. The story of any one is typical. Let Jim Long tell his own story.

"Up to two years ago, I worked on the farm. I didn't make much money so I jumped at the chance to get a job at this new factory. My family moved to town."

"What do you do in the factory?"

"It is my job to work in the galvanizing room where mostly I dip buckets, cans, chicken feeders and all sorts of things like that into a big pot of melted zinc, which is covered over with a foamy layer of some chemical."

"How many other people work in this department?"

"About twenty of us work right around the galvanizing pots, but there is another twenty in the same room doing other jobs, like cleaning up and pickling the metal before dipping, and stacking up stuff after we dip it."

"Do you ever get sick?"

"Not on the job, but two or three nights every week I get a peculiar sickness and nearly every other man working over the pot gets the same sickness. Some of the other men in the room get sick too, but not as regularly as we do."

"Can you tell ahead of time when you're going to be sick?"

"Not always, but there are certain days that we know we are more likely to be sick. These are rainy days, or days when it is snowy or foggy. Another time is usually on Monday or any other day when work has been shut down for a day or two. The more we rest up the better the chances we will be sick. That seems mighty peculiar to me."

"Now, tell me just how are you sick? When does it begin and what happens?

"Nothing much happens here at the plant, but after I get home, 'long about seven o'clock, the first thing that I know is that I get a terrible thirst. I try drinking water and that doesn't do any good. Then I think maybe lemonade would help, but that doesn't do the job. I never drank much liquor in my life until I came here, but with the terrible thirst I'd try drinking anything. I got to drinking beer and then whiskey. That would do a little good, but not much. I have spent a lot of money for liquor — more than I oughta. Long about nine o'clock I begin to get cold and shake all over. I go to bed and my wife covers me up with five and six quilts. Still I'm cold. I shake until you can hear the bed rattle. Some folks say that we all have chills and fever from mosquitos, like in malaria, but I never heard of any chills and fever in these parts except among these men at the plant. Maybe we caught it from each other, but nobody but us in the galvanizing room caught the disease. Nobody in the paint room has chills and fever and nobody in the office."

"Then what happens?"

"I keep on shaking until pretty near midnight and then I'm so tired that, chill or no chill, I get off to sleep. With all that cover, I

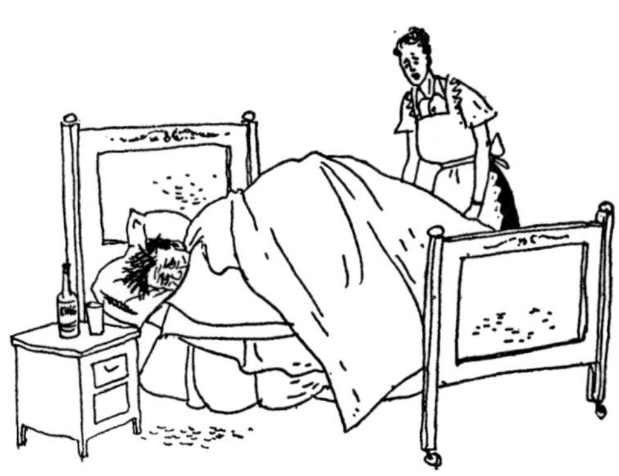

sweat like an old time drayhorse. The next morning when I wake up I think I'll never be able to work again. I'm as limp as a wet bathing suit. I have got a taste in my mouth like a manure pile on the farm. Just thinking about food makes me want to puke. My stomach is all upset and sometimes I cough. Every other man has just the same sort of trouble, and it's funny, but we all get sick pretty much on the same nights. After I stir around a while in the house, I feel all right, but don't eat much breakfast. By the time I get to the factory I feel good, put in a hard day's work, but maybe again that night or maybe not for three or four nights will I have any trouble — then it is always the same. Thirsty, chills, sweating, weakness."

All of this was very characteristic. This picture is typical of a well-known occupational disease — "zinc chills," "metal fume fever," "foundry fever," "brass workers' ague."

That night I spent in the home of the factory manager, who was grateful for my interest in his troubles. During the evening we visited a half dozen workmen. Unfortunately for them, but luckily for my objectives, two of them were in the throes of this bizarre affection. They were alarmed and their wives disturbed. To them it was explained that hot milk was the best agent for slaking their parched throats — not beer, not whiskey. From the doctor's point of view, no more evidence was needed. The condition was clear-cut.

The next morning, at the factory office, a conference was held. It was explained that some molten metals, such as in brass foundries, chandelier works, and galvanizing operations, give off fumes which when breathed by workmen produce a temporary disease without any chronic form, closely resembling malaria, but associated with pathologic thirst. On bright clear days, this fume more readily rises and is discharged through roof openings, but on rainy, foggy days the tendency is for this fume to hang low in a factory and thus workers are doubly exposed. If by accident the temperature of the molten metal is permitted to become higher than necessary, the likelihood of trouble increases because more fume is emitted. Old timers, particularly in the galvanizing trade, have a term for excessive temperatures. They speak of "burning the metal." Whenever this occurs, large numbers of exposed workmen may become involved during the ensuing night.

At this point, the somewhat incredulous plant engineer, a little resentful that any doctor should be taking a hand in the plant operations, sought to trip me up by inquiring, "Doctor, how do you account for the fact that on Monday night these men after having a good rest over Saturday and Sunday are almost sure to get sick. I think that what they do at home — overeating and drinking bad liquor over the week-end is what makes them sick and that the work has nothing to do with it."

For this I had an exact and ready explanation.

"For unknown reasons, men who are continually exposed build up some degree of tolerance. This tolerance is lost in as little as two days' time. After any absence, such as a vacation or an account of sickness or even over a week-end, whatever built up protection exists may be lost. It must have been your experience that any new workman on the first day of his employment usually is involved."

Reluctantly he agreed that this was true.

The factory manager, my unexpected host and new employer, then entered the conversation.

"Doctor, we are mighty glad you came to this town even if it was by accident. A lot of the good ladies around here feel pretty badly about us. Some of them would like to run us out of town. Of course, they can't do that. We have wanted to have the good will of everybody in this community, but it looks like we've got some of them down on us. So far you've told us only what's causing all this ruckus. Now can you tell us what we ought to do to stop these zinc chills?"

Here was my cue. I suggested the prompt installation of thermostatic control for the zinc pots so that the temperature of the metal would never rise above the minimum required for galvanizing. Then I urged that the fluff of foamy ammonium chloride floating on top of the molten zinc be increased in thickness, because this layer of another chemical prevents the escape of zinc fume.

Then I sketched in rough fashion an exhaust system with intakes to be located at the edge of three sides of the rectangular galvanizing pots. For especially bad days, when the fume was "high," I recommended that the galvanizers wear filter respirators of a type that would strain out the offending zinc oxide. Insurance was given that if all these things were done there would be no more sickness, and that after all the plant might be accorded respectability in the community.

"After all," said the manager, "these changes are fairly simple. If this is going to get rid of the disease, let's start today."

Later, a gracious letter confirmed my prediction.

No opportunity ever came to me to survey the subsequent state of sobriety in the working population of Barron. It is not known that the good ladies of the community hold further meetings in the Calvary Methodist Church, designed to uplift the moral tone of the village. It is not known that they realize that the accidental carrying of my baggage to their church meeting was any factor in righting an obvious wrong. But if all the facts were apparent, possibly these good ladies might accept me as the answer to their prayers.

Chapter 37

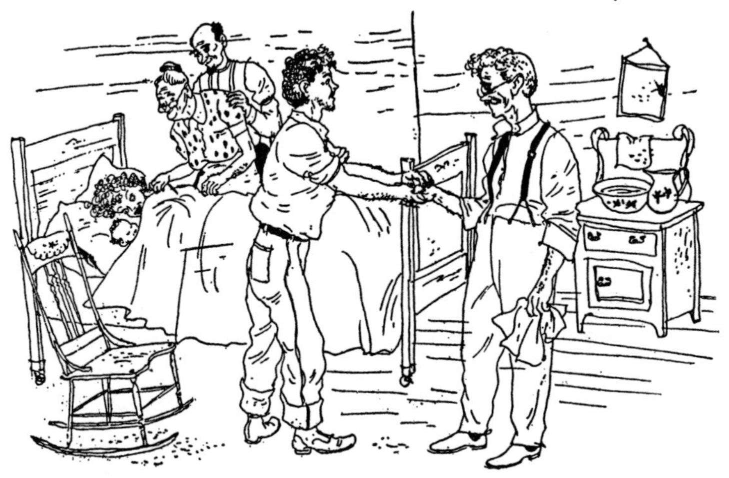

The Country Doctor Shows Up the Expert

THE RIGHTEOUS always get it in the neck — this inelegant adage may have been devised for the country practitioner of medicine. A member of this lusty race of man may start his day at four A.M. delivering a baby, shortly thereafter removing a pair of tonsils, repairing a hernia, examining school children as the morning wears on, making a hurried trip to the hospital in the county seat, thence the round of his patients, perhaps setting a broken leg, then holding office hours and ending the hectic day by delivering another baby.

In the meanwhile he may have been berated by some ungracious patient protesting a charge of three dollars for a fifteen mile trip into the country, or have occasioned discontent by refusing to step out of his role and treat sick calves. A family may have become grievously outraged when he failed to save the life of eighty-seven year old grandma who had been suffering from cancer for two years, or instead the wrath of the patient with blood pressure of two hundred and twenty may have fallen upon him, owing to his refusal to certify the man in perfect physical condition on an insurance application.

No less, the country doctor is not without his victories. One triumphed over me, and I, despite my tender ego, could but glory in his unostentatious conquest.

On a Tuesday following a Monday holiday, the country doctor paid our factory a visit as the guest of his son who worked in the medical department. The son had been anxious to exhibit the smooth modern efficiency of our department, and explain some of the recent scientific aids the plant had installed. His father was duly impressed by polarographs, potentiometers, nephelometers, spectographic microscopes, combustible gas indicators, interferometers. He admired all, understood none.

The day following a summer holiday, especially a Monday holiday, means a welter of work for the medical department of any factory. Always there is the crop of poison ivy victims, the inevitable sunburns, usually several exhausted workers having driven all night at the risk of their lives to be at the work-bench on time, and invariably the sufferers from hangovers.

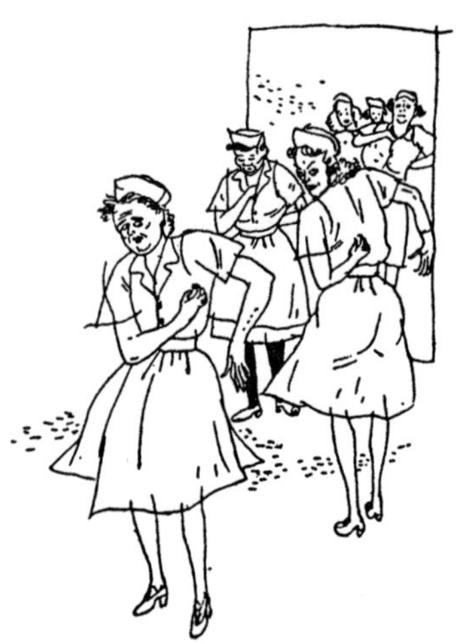

In our clinical section that Tuesday we had all of this and a bit of the unknown added.

Sixteen women had come to us in panic, itching, scratching, annoyed and frightened. All were suffering from numerous fiery red welts under shoulder straps, brassiere bands, waist bands and wherever else garments fitted tightly about their bodies. There were accusations of poison in the work material, and uncomfortable suspicions that some one of their number had brought in some dread disease, the latter less audibly charged and more widely believed. Each woman, innocent herself, blamed the others.

It was a bad situation, and my job to find its cause. Obviously it was related to some common factor in the small group all employed in a single workroom, but what?

No work materials could be blamed this time. The operations involved were the simple duties of packaging small steel parts for shipment. Insects then? Remembering the places of the welts it seemed inevitable that these were insect bites, yet what insect? It would be an ambitious mosquito indeed who would elect to do her blood sucking from beneath a lady's girdle; besides no mosquitoes were seen. If bedbugs were the offenders, they are no hit and run animals and someone would have detected their presence. Fleas have similar habits, and no one found any fleas. Chiggers or jiggers would establish their base of supply and settle down for long feasts. What possible insect might be expected to bite or sting under cover, then leave without a trace? A bite without an insect, a rash without an irritant.

"What the hell . . ." I muttered, easing away from the milling afflicted, now liberally plastered with itch-relieving medicaments. Every story had been heard, questions asked. What had they drunk? Were there any new materials in the department? With what were they cleansing their skins? No two patients came from the same residence.

Nearly every decade of adult life was represented. There were at least five races affected, a negress being among the sufferers, her race one that rarely incurs dermatitis.

We caught one lead. During the holiday period a vermin exterminator had been called in to apply roach powder in the women's wash rooms on this department's floor. All of the women involved frequented one of these washrooms and their work clothes hung in the same area. Here seemed the possible common denominator. Here it seemed until one man, a little abashed in the midst of so many women, had made his way through the throng to exhibit the same ailment.

With dampened enthusiasm we collected a sample of the insecticide and a spot analysis was made. Bad luck attended the process, for a trace of mercury was found which seemed to give plausibility to the matter — mercury dermatitis. Yet the pieces of the story failed to make an intelligent whole. Mercury dermatitis does not lead to marked itching; other washrooms had been treated and their users were not involved; furthermore, unused lots of the insecticide contained no mercury at all. Investigation proved that the boards making up the washroom had been treated with a mercury compound at the producing sawmill to prevent mildew, but this had been done years earlier. This lead had a dead end.

The country doctor wandered in.

"Doctor, what is this?" I asked him conversationally.

I beckoned to one of the afflicted factory workers, a small Italian woman. She walked cautiously over to us.

He looked briefly at the welts on the woman's wrists, shoulders, at the swollen redness on her chest. "Don't you really recognize this?" he asked incredulously.

"No," I replied shortly, wondering what hole in my education was about to be exposed.

"Well," he drawled, "I don't know much about factory diseases, but out in the country I see a lot of this every year. The farmers call it 'harvest itch,' 'threshers' itch,' 'farmers' itch,' 'straw itch,' sometimes 'grain itch.' " He chuckled at my puzzled expression. "It's caused by a small mite that lives on straw. Mostly occurs in summer. Pediculoides ventricosus, scientifically."

"Oh," I said watching my descent from a pedestal mirrored in the Italian woman's eyes.

"When the hired man sleeps on a straw-filled bedtick in winter, it often shows up. Then it's 'mattress itch.' " He spoke with unquestionable authority. "You must be doing some of the packing in straw," he suggested. Investigation proved that no packing in straw was being done in the department which housed the itch. Thus half the problem was solved. The other half, the source of the insects still was before us — my country consultant and me.

"Of course, Doctor," I remarked banteringly, "whenever we have medical visitors here we stage some demonstration within their own field. Next week we have a party coming up from Brazil. We hope to bring forth an epidemic of tropical disease just as we staged this for you."

He grinned and went to work. The first patients and others later affected in the department were all requestioned. "Were you in the country yesterday? Did you pitch hay? Were you in barns? Do you bed down rabbits in straw? Have you been on a fishing trip? Have you slept on a straw tick?"

In bland astonishment each successive worker denied all such acts. It was my confrere's turn to look puzzled. Somebody must have worked in that department yesterday, we decided. Hours had passed. Armed with itch-relieving medicaments, the patients were sent home. The work shift changed. I called in the chief of plant protection.

"Did anybody work in export packaging yesterday?" I asked him.

"Not a soul," was the quick reply.

"No one in the place at all, Chief?" I probed.

"Well," he remembered, "Well, yes there was. One night shift girl forgot it was a holiday, just coming in from her vacation."

"Go on, go on," I urged impatiently.

He looked surprised, but continued. "She brought her work clothes with her. Wanted us to keep them overnight so she wouldn't have to take them home. Couldn't keep 'em at the gate house so I let her leave 'em up in the washroom."

"That's it," the country doctor exploded. "That's our baby."

I nodded. "That girl is just about coming into the plant now. Chief, can you get her on the phone?" I queried. "Can you have one of your men steer her in here?"

"She had liquor in those clothes?" he asked, suddenly injured.

"Not liquor, Chief, just pediculoides ventricosus."

"No!" he said, amazed.

"Pediculoides ventricosus," my country colleague repeated.

The chief put in his telephone call and then turned back to us. "Doctor, I know I'm not supposed to ask questions, but even the old police chief ought to know a little about what's going on. Is there another pet skunk loose in the plant?" He looked unhappily from one to the other of us. At that point the girl in the case entered, preventing allayment of the chief's fears. He left.

Hopefully we turned our attention to her, but to our disappointment she did not enter scratching, or in any other way giving indication of being troubled. She was tall, dark complexioned naturally, and deeply tanned.

"You've just returned from a vacation?" we inquired.

"Yes — yesterday," she replied.

"Been on a farm, maybe?" the country doctor questioned.

"Why yes, I was," she told him, surprised.

And so it went — yes, she had worn her factory clothes around the farm; yes, she had rolled in straw stacks; yes, she had been much in the sun, but no sunburn because she had diligently applied skin tanning oil; yes, she had worn her work clothes at the farm and brought them back to work yesterday, and yes, she had hung them in the washroom. No indeed, she had no traces of skin disease.

Mentioning skin disease apparently reminded her of something. "Doctor," she said confidentially, "Doctor, I met one of the girls in my department coming in, and she says some of the women have a bad skin disease. I just want to tell you that those women on the first shift are a dirty lot. Do you think I'm apt to get something from them?"

"No, young lady," I told her. "I don't think there's a chance."

So once more we had a complete picture, a fitting of all the pieces, a fitting as precise as the seeds of a pomegranate. In utter guilelessness she had brought some thousands of harvest mites into the plant on her garments. Innocently, she had made the best possible arrangement for the mites to travel to every girl's garments . . . and they did. Equally innocently had she coated her own skin with the most effective armor against the plague — oil. It all fitted.

"Yes, indeed," I assured her confidently, "I believe you'll be quite safe from those 'dirty women.' "

Later the country doctor confided to his well-pleased son, "If that's the sort of thing that goes on in factories, maybe I can get a job."

To him I make definite reply, "Any time, Doctor, the job is yours. You take over the skin department."

Chapter 38

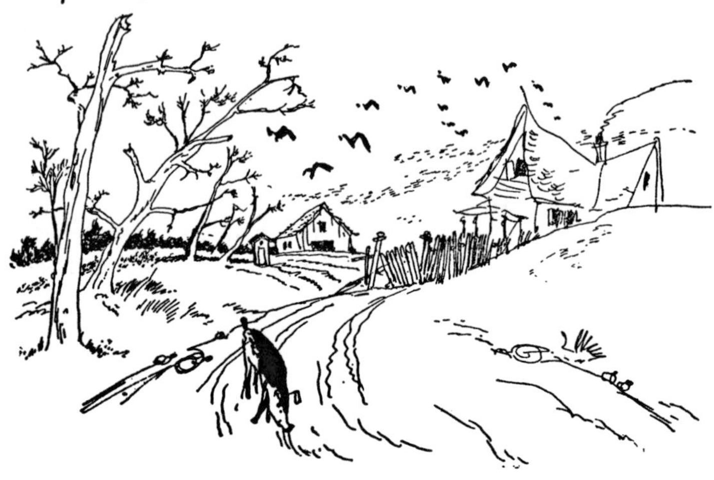

Fits from the Furnace

IN THE one general store in the small town of Bethlehem, I sought the location of the home of Dan Whitfield. The one clerk and two loiterers dallied a bit as glances were exchanged among the three of them. The clerk assumed the responsibility, but only hesitatingly replied,

"He comes in here every once in a while. We all know where he lives, but he's a pretty ugly customer and I wouldn't advise you to go huntin' him up unless you're sort of anxious about it. He's threatened to kill anybody that comes on his place. He isn't exactly hidin' out, but the law has been tryin' to put four or five of his kids in homes. The way those Whitfields live ain't fit for cattle. If he knew you were comin' and didn't know who you were, the whole kit of them would hide out in the woods 'til they were sure you were gone. If you go out there don't take any papers and don't take any gun unless you're willin' to get into a shootin' match."

"Doesn't sound very promising," I injected. "I wouldn't be very good in a shooting match, but, after all, my only mission is to arrange for Whitfield to get some money. If you'll tell me how to get there, I'll move on."

"Go east on this highway to the first crossroad, turn right and go about three miles until you come to Caney Road. Drive left on this road for about a mile until you see a big abandoned apple orchard and about in the middle of it the chimney of a burnt house. There's a little road there which maybe you can get over in your car. This ends up at a terrible old house at the foot of the hill, but you can't see this house from the orchard. That's were Dan Whitfield lives, with about ten skinny, trashy children and his wife. Good luck, mister."

As I drove along, dreading my mission, and frankly just a little scared, I reviewed what the insurance company had written me.

> "Six years ago this patient was injured in connection with some exposure on the inside of a hot steel furnace under repair. He did not have good treatment, and shortly after his initial injury began to have epileptic seizures. The Industrial Commission adjudged him temporarily totally disabled and, on their order, we have been paying him intermittently the full award. We have no unwillingness to continue these payments, but we have no medical information that he is still totally disabled and have experienced marked difficulty in keeping in touch with his whereabouts. He has lived in at least twenty backwoods communities in the past five years, has lived in at least four states. There are several warrants for his arrest for theft, neglect of family, destruction of property, assault and rumors of murders.
>
> "The last word we have about this beneficiary is that he is about thirty-five miles north of your city on the outskirts of the town of Bethlehem. Will you please attempt to locate this beneficiary and advise us as to his present condition and, if possible, procure a complete story of his original injury which we have never been able to obtain in satisfactory fashion?"

By this time I was at the tragically neglected apple orchard which in another day must have been a fine one. The soft April earth of the neglected road made driving precarious, but I wanted the car to serve as a noisemaker, in order that my approach might have no semblance of surreptitiousness. I elected to take the car along, but stopped one hundred yards away from the disreputable house, forsaken by its owners and undoubtedly no source of revenue from its present occupants.

A friendly razor-back hog, rooting up earthworms and grubs welcomed me, but did not miss a single stroke of rooting. I gathered that plentiful worms might be the sole item of his porcine diet. I wondered how this hog had fared when the ground was frozen. The marvel was that he had escaped the pot of his hand-to-mouth owners. It might have been suspected that this pig was a new arrival and possibly by the theft route.

Like a tail-wagging dog, I stood at my car and tooted a number of times, but excited nothing but a few crows nearby. Up at the house the steps had been torn away, probably for firewood, although wood was abundant in surrounding forests. I rapped on the door's lower panels. There was no response. Indiscreetly I peered through a closed window, there being no semblance of shade or curtain.

Huddled up in one corner, trying to make themselves invisible, were six naked children. Trying to shrink into nothingness, these six marasmic children hugged the wall and each other, flattened out like two rows of fish scales. No piece of furniture, not even a bench, was in this room.

After more knocking and more silence, I gave up the fight and started toward my car. Then it was I saw the gaunt, ill-kept man, leaning against a door jamb of the ramshackle barn. His right arm was not visible.

I knew at once that this was Dan Whitfield and that his hidden right hand was fingering his gun.

He undoubtedly had seen me peering through the window, and altogether he was not a reassuring sight. It was my cue to be ingratiating. Coldly he demanded,

"What do you want?"

It was no moment to start at the beginning. My next few words probably would determine some action with that hidden right arm.

Politely I said, "Mr. Whitfield, I may have some money for you in a few days."

The right arm dropped to his side and his body limbered up perceptibly. "Hell," he said, "I thought you were another one of them court agents tryin' to take my chillun away from me. They've run me out of nearin' ten places in Kaintucky and Indiany. They kept such good track of me that I was beginnin' to figure that the insurance company was in cahoots with 'em and was givin' 'em my backin' (address). For the past six months I ain't let the insurance company know where I was livin', but lately we all got so porely that I jest had to write 'em, but I ain't got any cash yet. Sure glad you've come."

Since Dan fast was building up the expectancy that I had money in hand for him, I hastened to explain,

"I'm just the insurance doctor. I came to talk things over with you a little bit and to fill out some papers, but since you may be a little hard pressed, I'm going to have a few dollars for you today."

Instead of his jaw dropping as I expected, his whole being registered complete satisfaction. One dollar evidently would have saved the day. Later on I gave him five dollars.

Then Dan became polite.

"Doctor," he said, "I ought ta be takin' you in the house, givin' you a good seat, and tellin' you to pull up to the fire, and I cain't do that. 'Bout all we got in the house is a fire. None of my chillun have been out of doors further'n the privy for more'n a month. Them young 'uns ain't got any clothes. My wife has got a kind of a dress, so we can go in the kitchen. We found a cook stove in this house when we come here two months ago, and I'll shake up a fire in it."

His wife was in the kitchen, sullen, suspicious and thoroughly pregnant. Dan moved his hand in her direction, saying, "My wife." I tried to better the situation by being especially pleasant. Even if she heard what I said, she made no reply, for at that moment there was a thumping of many bare feet, as the six children rushed upstairs, evidently having decided that their time had come and that they

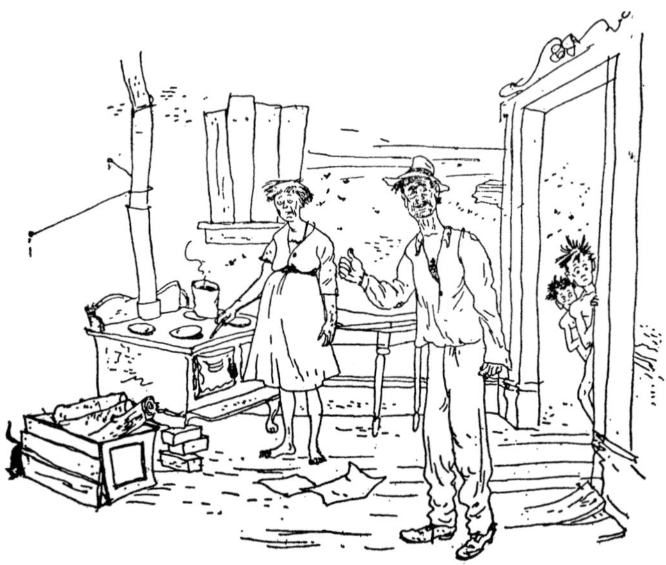

would make their last stand from that strategic point. The lack of all clothes prevented any rush to the outdoors. Dan started up the fire while I went back to the car to get my papers. Sitting on a pile of stovewood, I began to ask many questions and to make many notes. Later, pieced together, Dan's story, as stated by him would run as follows:

"'Long about seven yar ago, I got this job at the public works (steel mill) at Craterville, bein' a carpenter's helper. Mostly I just toted planks for the carpenters workin' on the company houses. We lived in one of them company houses. After a while I was put on the inside gang and did a little carpenterin' myself. One day about six yar ago, I fergit the exact time, but all that's been writ up on papers made out for the insurance company, the roof of one of the steel furnaces caved in when the company was awful busy and they wanted it fixed right then. It was all red hot in there so we waited a couple of days and it still was so hot that your clothes would smoke if you went in. The brick masons dug out the fallen-in part. Then we had to build a scaffol' for the masons to stand on to fix up the busted-down part. Six of us were workin'. We would take a deep breath and rush in with a plank with the nails already driv' through and give a couple of good plunks. We'd done wet our clothes, else they might have burnt off'n us. They were steamy as it was. All the lumber was soaked and that was steamy too. With six of us workin,' sometimes in twos, and sometimes just us, we knocked up that scaffol' pretty fast, but even at that it took about three hours — it wouldn't took more than half an hour workin' out in the open.

"We six started workin' nigh on to two o'clock. Along about five, I was all petered out and the rest of the boys too, but I was worse petered than them. All of a sudden I begin to see bright lights and red colors floatin' in front of my eyes and then things all went black, then I didn't know nothin'. From that time on, all I'm tellin' you is what other folks told me afterwards. They say that I acted crazy like for a while, yellin' and fightin' and then I dropped. They poured buckets of water on me cause they thought I had fainted. They just let me lie there for more'n an hour because they thought every minute I'd come to and go back to work. Long about half-past six, when they was through and goin' home, they took me across the road to a shack where some of the other boys bached and put me on a bed.

"They still figgered I ought to be all right soon, but when my wife come down, she was skeered foolish and told 'em to get the company doctor. There was no company doctor at that mill so they had to send over to the next town where there was another mill and where the company doctor lived. When the doctor come over, he took my fever and told my wife it was a hundred and seven. They wrung out blankets in cold well water and rolled me up in 'em and kept me that way all night. I didn't know nuthin' until pretty near sundown next day. Then I got brain fever and they couldn't move me away from that bach shack for three weeks. I guess I pretty near kicked the bucket. After I thought I was all well, I still wasn't. I begun to have these fits, foamin' at the mouth like a mad dog and all that. These fits come on me 'round ever two weeks, made no difference where I was, in bed, at the store, on the road, anywhere. Sometimes I'd hurt myself. The company wouldn't ever let me go back to work. They give my family a chance to get grub at the commissary, but no money. After I started to be better, they made out a lot of papers and there was lawyers and courtin', but my lawyer made them fork over back money and they signed up writin' to give me more money right along. The company made me move out of the company house so I had to go back down in the country. Pretty soon a lot of folks got to messin' in about my chillun. They took me into court and got some sort of right to take away my chillun. Those chillun are mine and nobody ain't goin' to take 'em away from me. No sir. Them times was only four. There's six now and another one comin'. From that time on, Doctor, there ain't been nothin' but misery. Me and my family movin' from settlement to settlement, nobody wantin' us, everythin' bad happenin' in them towns blamed on me, no vittles, no clothes, no money. For a while I lost the backin' of the insurance company which is why I didn't get no money. Half the time some young un sick, my wife porely all the time and me havin' fits. What else do you want to know doctor?"

There were many things I wanted to know.

"How often are the seizures occurring now? Can you tell when the seizures are coming on? Do you think you're getting better or worse? Do you want any money sent here to this address? You can be sure that I will not tell anyone of the plight of your family if you forbid, but it will be mighty easy to get some food in the house and some clothes for your children."

I made my medical examination as best I could in that bare kitchen. The only utensil I saw was a big wooden dough tray smeared over with smelly sour dough. I had to turn my back on this to keep from gagging as I went about my examination. There were the customary telltale markings of recent epileptic seizures — scars on a bitten tongue. Apart from an epileptic, thoroughly scarred up tongues are a rarity.

Too, it seemed quite obvious that both this man and his wife were frankly feeble-minded. It was a safe guess that some of the cringing children also were feeble-minded. The prospects for the one soon to be born certainly were not comforting.

All of the medical portions of the story related by Dan already were well authenticated. My own medical examination, inadequate as it was, furnished conviction that epileptic seizures were occurring still, even though at wider intervals. This patient's injury at the steel mill manifestly was not "sunstroke" nor "heat exhaustion." Clearly it was a case of "thermic fever," the indoor equivalent of sunstroke and foremostly due to the excessive temperatures within the caved-in furnace unit.

There could be no question about the actuality of an initial injury. That epileptic attacks may appear for the first time after such an injury is possible, although not frequent. Fortunately for my peace of mind, this decision already had been made by a court.

This court rightly or wrongly had decided that Dan's epilepsy was inaugurated by his injury. My professional integrity was fortunately not put to a test.

Even if there had been no signs of continued impairment, even if Dan had insisted that he was hale and hearty, free from all distress, I would have been tempted to urge the insurance company to send all moneys then due, to send them promptly, and to plan to send more until their maximum legal responsibility had been fulfilled.

All this I promised Dan and his tattered, bedraggled wife and away I went. Looking over my shoulder, and through the upstairs windows, I saw six pair of eyes—six wasted, wistful faces. Ahead of me the still rooting hog gave a low grunt of delight—I was not sure that this resulted from the finding of an extra-large grub or in approval of this adventuring physician finishing up a disagreeable assignment.

As the motor began to turn, out dashed Dan from the kitchen, waving my five dollar bill. "Wait, Doc, wait. Do you care if I ride back in town with you? I want to get some grub for the young uns. They ain't et rightly since I recollect."

Maybe Dan gave thought to his own empty belly as well. If so, with reason, and with my sanction.

Chapter 39

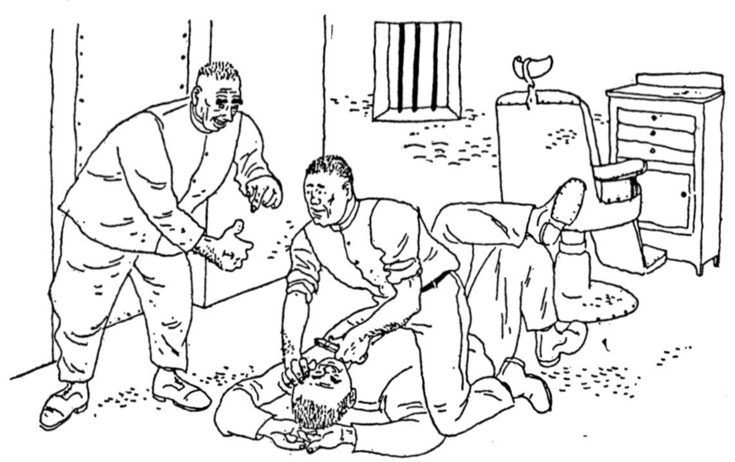

The Workers' Crotchets and Incubuses

TO THE everlasting discredit of a lot of people who hold themselves as being of a finer stripe than laborers, is their belief that somehow or other these toilers are far less subject to physical or mental pain than is their own lot. They, who shoutingly demand novocaine before they permit their dentist to go about drilling for the smallest cavity, see no reason why a workman should have that same novocaine for the amputation of a finger.

There is a scant evidence that any group of normal beings is much less sensitive to pain than others. Some persons well familiar with pain endure real pain more quietly than others. For some abnormal men and women the situation may be different.

As a young physician doing a temporary stint of medical work in a state penitentiary where medical services were of the lowest order, I was called upon to extract a tooth in a big burly murderer. Without experience or great strength I went about the job wretchedly. For a half hour I wrestled with that tooth, prying, jerking, but it didn't budge. The pain, I thought, must have been horrible. I apologized. The amiable prisoner was all smiles. He beamed, "I like to have my gums massaged that way." A hospital orderly, likewise a prisoner, stronger than I and wiser in prison dentistry, took over the job. First he climbed up onto the lap of the murderer to gain leverage, and then with the patient flat on the floor he essayed some new maneuvers. There still was no loss of tooth. Another waiting patient entered this dental arena. He was a giant with a half-amputated thumb. That thumb stub was as large in diameter as a child's forearm. He explained, "If I kin git this here 'nub' of mine for a lever, I kin pull that tooth."

That was successful, but there was plenty of gore. The complacent patient who, I thought, should have been pardoned for extraordinary heroism, merely noted, "Down below, on the other side is another bad one. Would you folks like to work on that one?"

Not proudly do I extoll that form of medicine. I suspect that that patient may have been pain deadened by central nervous system syphilis but I have no proof. He was the abnormal exception. Those who fatuously believe that all workers have been shorn of half their nerves of sensation, need to have the scales beaten off their own minds.

These same silly ones likewise may believe that the mental and emotional equipment of industrial workers is irresponsive to the shocks, stresses and strains that bring about the quirks and kinks in the affairs of these self-styled "superior" beings. It may be true that only the elite may afford to indulge in the luxury of psychoanalysis and face a two-thousand dollar bill for this service, but in spite of the saving grace of long hours of toil, a high percentage of workers everywhere are handicapped by a world of neuroses — their own and those of their fellows.

The industrial worker is highly vulnerable to the buffeting in his world. Like most of the rest of us, he is beset by uncertainties, anxieties, insecurity, inferiority, phobias, neuroses, fear of not fitting into his group, fear that he may be disliked, a little insecure as to his job, uncertain about the attitude of his foreman toward him, disturbed by troubles at home, a complaining wife, demanding children. His work world may be filled with noise, monotony, fatigue.

For many, shortened hours of labor, however gladly accepted, only add to the burden of the worker's living. Scant opportunity for recreation, unattractive homes, few friends, limited satisfaction. Deeply hidden in the average workman are lonesomeness and anxiety.

During those months that I devoted to a certain investigation of ulcers of the stomach and intestines due to zinc sulfate, my prize patient, a galvanizer, was not fully cooperative. Maybe I should not blame him for objecting to the downing of a pint of tasteless, thickish barium sulfate in order to make his stomach outlines stand out in an x-ray film. At any rate, this patient, Claud Sykes, too often stayed away just when I needed him. Regularly I had to drive down back streets, narrow alleys, to a tenement hovel and there climb up three flights of stairs to be greeted by an apologetic Claud who regularly overplayed his symptoms in an effort to justify his non-cooperation.

My first visit to Claud's home was the enlightening one. Out in the middle of the one big room was a motley pile of bones—steak T-bones, backbones, bones from pork chops, ham bones, and here and there small bones which, my guess would be, came from pigs' feet. All of these bones were thrown about in artless fashion, so as to give the impression of the casual. At first I kept quiet about them, believing that they might be related to some religious belief or practice, some cultist affair to which Claud's ignorant mind readily might have been bent.

As the hour passed along, and a little more friendliness appeared, I inquired, "What are all the bones for?"

My curiosity had been brought to this point by observing under one or more of the beds in the room additional bones.

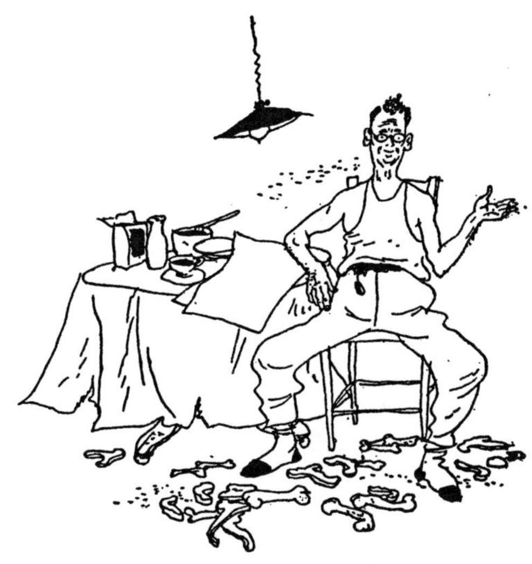

Quite sincere was Claud's reply, "Doc, we just want folks to know that we have good eatin' around this place. If they see these bones here anybody that comes in the house can see that we live high. Thick steaks, ham bones, spareribs, rabbit bones, everything. If it wasn't for these bones here in the house, folks that come around might think we were just ordinary trash. We ain't trash. Look at them bones."

Then I asked, "Well, what about these other bones under the bed?"

"Sometimes when we know folks are coming that we don't like we just put out more bones to make them mad. They probably don't have good grub at their house, and when they see all these bones that we are able to lay out here, that puts them just in the place they ought to be in."

Apparently, since only a portion of the evidences of past delicacies were tossed out at my coming, I must perforce believe either that there was no need to impress me or, perhaps, this curtailment was due to my warning as to proper diet and the avoidance of meat.

Here then is a workman utterly inadequate in his feelings toward the world, in his appraisal of himself, seeking to build up social prestige through the hoarding of evidence of past feasts—held as tangible proof that they were not the sort of family that would live on sow belly and corn bread.

This story will be labeled as fantastic, but it represents a precise recital of the sort of quirks that tangle up the lives of many thousands of workmen.

Throughout all industry, the greatest single need in terms of new departures may be found in the realm of neuroses. Not one industrial plant in a hundred employs a psychologist or a psychiatrist. Mental hygiene, while often knocking on the door of industry, rarely has been admitted.

A recent issue of a medical journal carried, under the fetching title "The Technique of Listening to the Worried Employee," a salutary article that includes this paragraph:

> "Psychoneurotics are emotionally immature individuals. In all these cases there is a definite fixation of the attention upon the patient himself and an emotional reaction far out of proportion to his difficulties. Too often his symptoms are a direct play for sympathy and attention, or an excellent alibi for failure in a given situation. These patients translate their disappointment and difficulties into physical symptoms much in the same manner that a young boy develops stomach ache early on the morning he has a difficult test at school. The grown-up is more adroit, and sometimes his pseudo-symptoms will triumph over even a laboratory checking."

For these unhappy workers, the continuous gnawings of work, fatigue, inferiority feelings, distrust, insecurity become the bases of chronic grouches, endless irritability, pseudo-disabilities, anti-social reactions, feelings of neglect and persecution.

Many a worker who in a strike situation has enlisted in what he believes to be some righteous cause in the procurement of workers' just dues, is, on better analysis, found to be striking only because at last he has attracted a little attention to himself, feels a little important, is given opportunity to talk, and has an audience.

With full recognition that this book is designed to interest rather than to teach, it still may be well to include here a few definitions appropriate to human whimsies. I have difficulty in forgetting that I am a teacher.

> "A NEUROSIS is an apparent affection of the body or mind without the existence of any organic change to account for the disease or abnormality.

Thus neuroses are functional and are not real. In common parlance, they represent imaginary diseases and are commonly related to emotional instability, mental quirks, discontent, etc.

"A NEUROTIC is a person with one or more neuroses.

"NEURASTHENIA is a state of a person with neuroses in which excessive fatigability plays a prominent role.

"A NEURASTHENIC is a person affected by neurasthenia.

"PSYCHASTHENIA is the state of a person with one or more neuroses in which anxieties and apprehensions play a prominent role.

"A PSYCHIASTHENIC is a person affected by psychasthenia."

THE most vivid portrayal of the material out of which neuroses are brought to the point of thriving comes from animal experiments, in which the uncertainties and insecurities within a dog's life made a thorough-going neurotic of a dog. In a small, dim room, a healthy dog was maintained under none too pleasant circumstances — a slim diet, no playing, no human companionship. The dog became lonesome, unhappy. Then, by arrangement, after the dog had become adjusted to his disagreeable environment, there was flashed on within the room a sizable circle of light. Promptly at a fixed time thereafter, such as one hour, a sumptuous dog meal was provided. Always the flashing on of this circle meant the coming of abundant food for a famished dog — no light, no food — no food without light. Over and over this was repeated until the dog himself accepted the coming of the light like approaching footsteps as the inevitable forerunner of food. The hungry dog in the interval between light and food drooled saliva, hopefully pranced up and down the room, awaiting the certainty of food.

Then came the time when also by arrangement on the opposite side of the room there was flashed a square of light of the same size and intensity as the circle. This square of light was the symbol of scanty food for a long period. Following the exposure of this light, twenty-four to thirty-six hours of bread and water became the regimen. This was distressing to the dog. He grumbled, sulked, slept, but he accepted the inevitable and came to know the square light meant no food.

Then came the time when under the experimental circumstances, both lights were flashed on the walls simultaneously. Here came the uncertainty, here came the perplexity, one light through long experience honestly promised food in a short time — another light heretofore honest in its meanings promised no food. Here was the dilemma — yes and no — food and no food. No wonder the poor dog went berserk.

In human life, a thousand similar situations confront the worker's life. Into one ear is shouted one thing and into the other the opposite. There is no definite right and no definite wrong. An endless need for choosing, selection, not always may the choice be made — the choice as made turns out to be wrong — hope becomes despair — promises turn into faithlessness — fond plans melt in the hands.

To assuage our topsy-turvy personal worlds, we create for ourselves neuroses. We return to childhood, we excite hidden traumas of infancy, we create imaginary ills or feckless mannerisms, all consciously or unconsciously to serve as scabs in the protection of raw mental surfaces.

It was my lot as a medical student to be included in a special group for the study of causes of accelerated immediate weight losses. When my time came, completely stripped of all clothing, I was stretched out on the bare surface of a giant balance as sensitive as the usual chemical laboratory scales. Through proper arrangement, a needle recorded on a blackened surface of a kymograph my slow, orderly, weight loss. I had been instructed to lie relaxed and comfortable and, as far as possible, thinking of nothing. Complying with this request as best I could, I overheard the professor in charge whisper to the third person in the room, a message apparently not intended for my ears.

The message was, "I'm glad to get this man on the scales today because he may not be in school after the end of this week. It is being rumored around among the faculty he's going to be dropped for unsatisfactory scholastic work."

Immediately down, down, down went the needle. My loss of weight accelerated by three times. Could this be true? Was my work bad? Could the faculty drop me? Why had I not been told? What work was so bad as all that? Was there any way to stop it?

Out of such material, neuroses if not created are well served. Of course, the professor's remark was made only to serve the purposes of his experiment. Off the scale and into my shorts, the professor readily dissipated my distress by laughingly telling me the truth. In all of life, there are too many distressing stimuli that are not followed by any offsetting remedial measure.

In a famous motion picture of a decade ago, centering about the harassments of industry and exaggerating them, the chief actor was caused to carry on stereotyped motions long after his work hour, but precisely following the work motion pattern. In this comedy film, this exaggeration was good clean fun. Some of us who viewed the film with more or less professional eyes overlooked the possibility that in real life the same thing may happen.

During one investigation in Illinois, it was my habit to stand unobtrusively near the main exit through which the majority of all workers passed at the end of the work shift. In general, I was looking for any evidences of obvious fatigue, for characteristic postural damage, and for other leads that might guide later investigation. Day by day my attention was attracted by three or four workers, all of whom were making the same motions and at the same rate and apparently all unbeknownst to them. Mentally this group was marked and their exact duties observed on subsequent days. Their motions as they walked down the street were a continuation of these same motions made a thousand times during the hours of employment. Under my very eyes, the exaggerations of the movie film had come to life.

In another plant, one workman of decades far beyond the draft age complained of inability to stand at his work, which faithfully he had performed over many years. His request was for another job or for some arrangement whereby he could do his present work seated. He insisted that his right leg had "gone bad" on him. His request led to a thorough medical examination. There was no evidence of any injury to the right leg, no atrophy, no breaking down of the foot arch, no nerve injury, no arthritis. This workman was assured that there was no determinable reason for his changing work and going to an inferior position. This advice was followed by a marked acceleration in the affection, until within a few weeks the right leg to all appearances was paralyzed. The workman gave up all duties, went about on crutches, hopeless, complaining. The plant physicians were baffled. A psychiatrist was called in and promptly reported the condition as spurious. "But of course," he added, "it is just as real to the patient as though it were organic. Behind this is something, but it is in the mind of this good workman. We owe it to him to find out."

The psychiatrist did find out. Then came the facts. The workman had a son of draft age of whom he was exceedingly fond and proud. None too patriotic, the father resented his country's taking away his son, for whom he had plans for education, to run the risks of warfare, camp diseases and the usual vicissitudes of the soldier. In his son's behalf, he had made vigorous claim before a draft board of a childhood injury to his son which he was sure would render him unfit for military service. This childhood injury as described affected the right leg. While in truth there may have been some injury at this earlier period, there were no genuine residual effects and the adoring father kindly but unmistakably was given to understand that his claims for the boy were to be given little credence.

There was the trauma. In resentment, the father, all unknown to himself, created within his own leg an injury that he may have honestly believed existed in the boy — sheer neurosis. A few months later when the boy returned home, discharged from military duty because of disturbing snoring, the father made a marvelous recovery. Naturally, whatever nostrum was in use at the time was accorded the accolade for the cure.

But aren't the facts apparent?

Even as for you and me, the toll of the worker's day often is represented by wholly needless crotchets. They, as you and I, translate these knots into headaches, diarrheas, gastric upsets, unnecessary fatigue, hatreds, and on through an endless lot of created ills behind which we attempt to hide our unhappiness, our discontent, our anxieties, our unwillingness to endure the blows of living.

When industrial hygiene attains to a full measure of its health conservation possibilities for workers, it will be found to embrace adequate consideration of the worker's mental and emotional processes as well as his fingers, toes, and eyes.

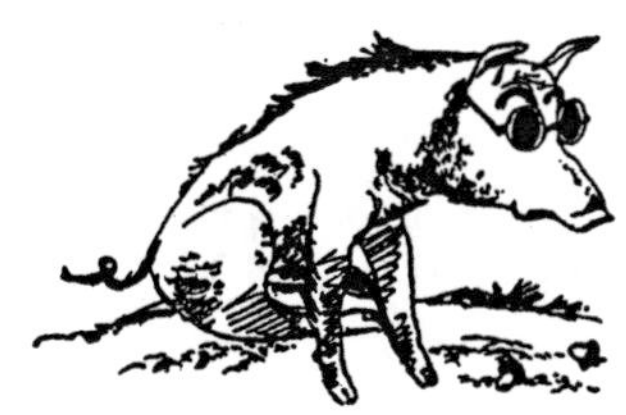

Chapter 40

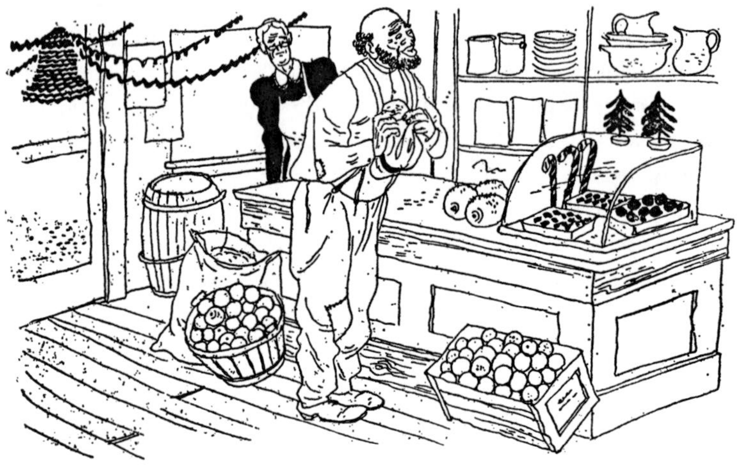

Uncle Jeff's Big Catch

SOME WORK materials may cause cancer. Over the years a long list of "carcinogenic" agents has accumulated. Most of these agents are complex derivatives of coal tar. A few chemicals pick out the urinary bladder as the point of attack; a larger number elect the skin as their site of damage.

In the United States, occupational cancer is so rare that, in a professional lifetime, I have seen not more than three cases, and these were of the "maybe" variety. This statement does not apply to cancers real and imaginary caused by repeated friction. With this latter sort, my first acquaintance was made at the age of eight — not that I was doing any precocious practice of medicine at the time. Actual diagnosis was deferred twenty years, and then it was not "occupational tumor."

Uncle Jeff was an old negro sharecropper on my grandfather's plantation. As he plowed with his one mule, his allotment of cotton land the plow lines were tied behind his waist to free his hand for grasp on the plow handles. Many summers of irritation of the plow lines rubbing against the hot skin may have been a factor in the growth of a large, fatty tumor — a lipoma.

These fat tumors are fairly common among all people, and by far the greater number certainly may not be associated with work as the cause. This class of new growths is benign, and in no sense may it be regarded as cancerous.

Uncle Jeff's tumor was enormous — the size of a cantaloupe and slightly pedicled, that is, it was on a stem. Even fifty years ago, medical science was so advanced that this tumor might have been removed with utter safety, but Uncle Jeff scorned all medical care.

He philosophized, "Gawd gib me dat big bunch fur er reason. If he didn't want me to haff it, he'd neber haff gib it tuh me. If he wants me to haff it, I keeps it and do the bes' I kin."

I, with the curiosity of any eight year old boy was anxious to see that tumor and pried around at every opportunity, but Uncle Jeff's pride always led to the bulge in his side being covered up. This pride got him into trouble with Miss Cora Watts, the new storekeeper of the one tiny country store in our little village.

It was Christmas time, with Christmas day only a little ahead. In the store there were cocoanuts, oranges, apples, new kinds of candy, and, most exciting of all, fireworks, for, in the South, Christmas is celebrated with fireworks and not the Fourth of July. Uncle Jeff had no money to buy these marvels, but no harm would be done if he just went down and looked at them. A look at other people's things was about all that Uncle Jeff got out of Christmas. Miss Cora was suspicious. She suspected all negroes as being thieves. She was a newcomer. Her eyes scarcely left harmless Uncle Jeff as he lingered over the strange wares. Having sated his eyes, if not his stomach, he shuffled toward the door with his stooped gaunt body, but his tumor stood out in bulging incrimination. Apparently outwitted, Miss Cora blocked his way at the door and yelled to the men passersby on the roadway, "Help, help! This thieving man has stolen my cocoanuts!"

There was a rush of several men to her aid. The outcry of any woman in those days against any negro would bring ready response. Trying to protect her property, Miss Cora grabbed hold of the tumor. It was soft and fleshy. No cocoanuts there. All of the men knew Uncle Jeff and about his tumor. As soon as they saw what was going on, all the men laughed, but Uncle Jeff cried and Miss Cora cried in her shame and embarrassment. To make amends, she gave a cocoanut to Uncle Jeff—maybe the only one he ever had.

When my grandfather heard of this, he was a little upset. He felt a little responsible, since he too believed that the rubbing of the plow line had caused the tumor. Uncle Jeff was called in and told that he need work no more on the farm, that he would be taken care of as long as he lived.

His new job was to look after me. He was in his second childhood —I in my first. We became playmates. Uncle Jeff knew where the best wild plums grew, where to dig bait for fishing, where the best fishing holes were, where the buzzards built their nest, where we might see a "possum" in a tree, how to build a raft. This lore brought happy days the following summer after Uncle Jeff's misfortune at Christmas time.

Early in the summer Uncle Jeff was troubled. He was "cogitatin'." He lived with his secret, drawing away a little from me. I felt lonesome and wanted to break over into whatever was occupying his mind.

Then came the day that he poured out a most exciting plan:

"Boy, we been doin' a passel of fishin', but we ain' doin' it right. We doan use no big hooks, and no big strings, and no big bait. We ketch plenty puny fish. No big fish gonna mess 'roun with just one worm no more'n you'd mess around with just one grain of rice. Out in this here crick there's plenty of water for powerful big fish to live. I'se been thinkin' that you and me oughta try to interest them big ones."

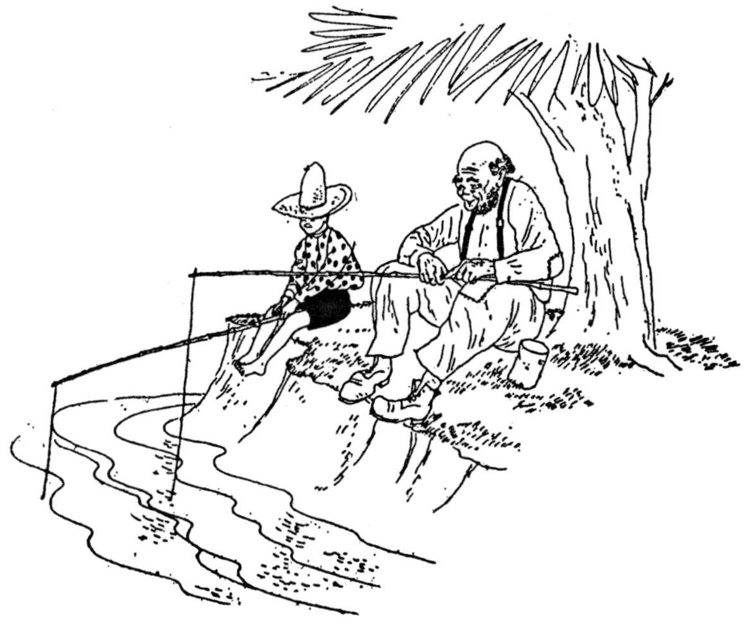

Here was a thought that both entranced and frightened an eight year old. Uncle Jeff's arguments completely convinced me. At once I wanted to know, "What will we use for bait? What kind of pole will be big enough? Where can we get a hook? How big do you think these big fish might be?"

Uncle Jeff's planning had included all these points.

"Fur bait we oughta use er chicken or er rabbit. A chicken is too good eating, so let's figger on a rabbit. In your grandpap's garden I seen a big rabbit night 'fore las' about sundown, eatin' on the pea vines. We'll git that rabbit. Fur a hook, that's caused me a lot of cogitatin'. Fust I thunk we could partly stretch out a big horse shoe, but den I recollected about your grandpap's well grabs. Them's the very thing. Dere's three prongs on the well grabs and an eyehole at the top."

"But, Uncle Jeff, what can we use for a line and pole?"

"Them ain' goin' to cause no trouble. We'll jest use a long piece of calf rope for the fishin' line and no pole a'tall. We'll kill the rabbit and stick him on the well grabs with the calf rope tied to it and then tie the rope to a big stout roof hanging over some deep place, then throw the rabbit out into the deep water. We'll do this at night kase the big fish doan do any traipsin' 'roun by daylight. They's night brutes like pant'ers and wild cats."

With great excitement, we set about these plans. All were easy except for the rabbit. Just before sunset we hid in the tall Johnson grass awaiting the arrival of the rabbit. Uncle Jeff had his antiquated single-barreled shotgun. His hands trembled nearly as much as mine. It was almost miraculous that he with his half-blinded eyes killed the rabbit, but he did. Here was gory bait which should entice the biggest of the creek's fishes. The well grabs with the rabbit tied on with binder twine duly were cast out into deep water.

In order that Uncle Jeff might wake me at four o'clock next morning, I laid out a pallet of two quilts on the piazza floor, as near to the steps as possible. Uncle Jeff went to his cabin by the big chestnut tree beyond the barn. No amount of excitement can keep an eight year old boy awake all night. I was soundly sleeping when Uncle Jeff shook me, saying,

"The time's come, boy — git up. Doan make much noise. You doan wanna wake the res' of the folks."

I was immediately ready. I had slept with all my clothes on.

Over the back fence into the apple orchard, across the rail fence into the cow pasture, through the barn lot fence, but Uncle Jeff couldn't keep up. His old legs were wobbly and his big tumor flopped up and down as he tried to run. He kept yelling,

"Wait for Uncle Jeff. He wants to see the big fish same as you does."

We went together through the buckeye bushes, through the catalpa brush, down to where the cane reeds blocked off any ready view of the water. I got a little ahead of Uncle Jeff and was standing in a little sandy clearing not more than forty feet away from the big tree where the calf rope was tied, but I couldn't see the water. Waiting for Uncle Jeff to catch up, I heard a terrible splashing. Uncle Jeff heard it too. The great moment had come. Both of us were scared. We were a little sorry that we had ever thought of this unprecedented enterprise. Why hadn't we left well enough alone and caught only small fish like other people? The thrashing around and splashing got even louder. Uncle Jeff then said,

"Boy, we's ketched him, but that noise sho do sound turrible big. I s'pect we orta pray. Let's get down on our knees."

Badly scared, we both did. Uncle Jeff began,

"Oh Lawd, this ole man and this lil white boy has done somethin' that mebbe we ortan to done. Nobody else Lawd evah thought of ketchin' great big fish out of this here crick. Mebbe 'taint natural, but Lawd we can hear him splashin' and thrashin'. If you hadn't wanted us to ketch it, you wouldn't haff let him get on the hook, so Lawd when we hear him out there like we does evah once in a while, we knows that you doan mind. Lawd, I ain't strong liken I usta be and dis here is an awful lil white boy. Iffen we gits in trouble with dis big fish, please Lawd remember these lumps over on my side and doan let us git in too much trouble. And Lawd iffen it looks to you like we's about to get in trouble, you jest let that big ole fish cut loose from them well grabs and git away. Lawd I'se scared but I hopes it's all right with youse. Amen."

I piped up my shrill "Amen" too.

Then we pushed back the cane, traveled for a few feet and there was Uncle Jeff's big catch.

During the night decomposition had set in and gas had formed in the rabbit's body, not that I knew that as a small boy. The bait with its well grabs had floated to the surface and then over into the shallow water, at the low bank, the watering place for the animals. Down had come my grandfather's old rangy sow for her early morning drink and wallow. The finding of the dead rabbit in shallow water was an unexpected porcine boon. Trying to tear off the morsels, handicapped by water, rope, twine and well grabs, the old sow hadn't managed it very well and right through her cheek she'd run one of the well grab's tines. She was hooked like any fish, but not too securely. With a woof of extra fright due to our presence, the bloody, mistreated indignant old sow luckily broke loose from the hook and disappeared through the brush.

A quivering and disappointed Uncle Jeff sat down in silence for a while, and then:

"I 'spect your grandpap's gwine to be right mad at what we's done to the old hog. Jest 'sposin we doan evah tell him nothin' about it? From now on, boy, mebbe you'd better do all the thinkin'. Mebbe dis here bunch in my side done pizened my brain so's that I kin think only foolish things."

Chapter 41

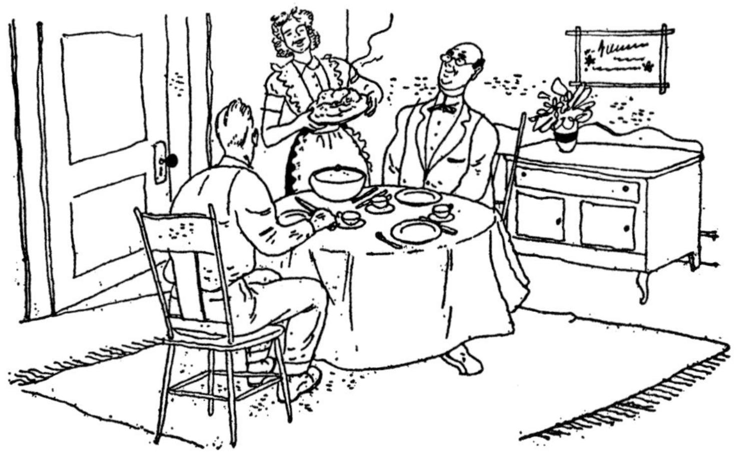

"Tet" and "Tri"

EVERY trade has its lingo. Most workers quickly reveal their trade by their language. Picturesqueness of industrial macaronics is excelled only by the argot of military forces. In the language of the workman that much used, gaudy material, red lead, is "catsup," but among the armed forces, real catsup becomes "red lead."

No term descriptive of a job is quite so appropriate as "tack spitter." This bit of St. Giles Greek marks the man or woman in the upholstery trade who, deftly tacking away, promotes efficiency with a mouthful of tacks, and a magnetic hammer. One by one the tacks are brought to proper position between the lips to be picked up by the hammer face — and the practice goes on day by day — year by year. Since the temptation is never resisted to show off one more example of occupational disease it may be noted that, in times past, lead-containing upholstery tacks occasionally sent the "tack spitter" to the hospital with lead colic.

Among many other thousands of workers the terms "tet" and "tri" are as common as "breakfast" and "supper." "Tet" is the vernacular for carbon tetrachloride, or tetrachlormethane, if you prefer that term, while "tri" is thieves' Latin for trichlorethylene. These agents are both friends and foes of mankind, but not under the same circumstances. Many millions of unwanted hookworms ruefully might trace their expulsion from the gastro-intestinal tract to carbon tetrachloride. This oily material, except among alcoholics, is almost harmless to human beings taken by mouth, but death to some parasites.

Breathed into the lungs in the form of its vapor and in large quantities, it is anything but friendly. In the lore of the pharmacology of "tet" it is recorded that large quantities of this substance harmlessly may be deposited in the stomachs of dogs in the quest for greater knowledge of its parasitic action but unfortunate is that dog that vomits. He may be killed by the "tet" vapors of his own vomitus. "Tri," or if we must be proper, trichlorethylene, is even more friendly. Inhaled in the form of its vapors and under proper circumstances, it is a well nigh perfect general anesthetic in some types of surgical operations, such as in the pregnant woman with tuberculosis who must be operated. Already so many hazards are being run that the risk of lung irritation from any anesthetic is most undesirable. Here is one opportunity for "tri" to serve a useful function in the conservation of mankind.

In industry "tet" and "tri" have other duties to perform. Both are "degreasers." In the many ramifications of the metal industry large numbers of workers appear to be working at cross purposes. One group day by day busily applies greases and oils to metals to keep down corrosion—to prevent rust. Another group, equally actively, goes about the business of removing every trace of oils and grease—this for such purposes as metal plating—both steps are necessary in the orderly flow of the work.

This seeming ridiculousness is what makes opportunity for jobs for the fifty-five million or more workers in this country. "Tet" and "tri" line up not with the "greasers" although they have been known so to do, but mostly with the "degreasers." Here, though, "tri" greatly outshines its cousin "tet" and has almost pre-empted the field, while "tet" has found its prime places of usefulness in fire extinguishers and the garment cleaning plant.

"Tri" in its unfriendlier moods does queer things to some workers, as in the well disguised instance now to be related.

In pre-war days there came to one of the manufacturing centers of prosperity Jim Robert Stevens and his wife Ella Mae. They came from Tennessee and that state's Sequatchie Valley, which name is said to mean "hog and hominy." Apparently all of the hog and hominy had been consumed, and Jim Robert and Ella Mae were not wholly unacquainted with poverty. In seeking prosperity they brought little with them save a profound religion of a kind sometimes unkindly associated with the Bible belt.

These young people were the sort that were likely to have hanging in their living room such mottos as "Christ is the Head of this House." On Sundays this devout pair found themselves in Sunday school where Jim Robert was the secretary and Ella Mae was the teacher of the primary class. During later church services Jim Robert took up the collection, and at least once a month the good pastor graced Ella Mae's meal of southern fried chicken. Over the small dining room table the three friends bemoaned the evils of the demon rum. It was out of just this alcoholic attitude that there came this semblance of tragedy.

These happy days were threatened with an abrupt end when one day, Ella Mae, more than a little dejected and sorrowful went to the preacher and reported:

"Brother, after all these years, and I sure hate to say it, I think Jim Robert has taken to drinkin'. Every night when he comes home from work he staggers around like any other drunk, red faced, shoutin' and yellin', doesn't quite know what he's doin'. I think he's stoppin' by some place between home and the mill and gettin' himself some liquor. He acts like any other drunk even to vomitin'.

There's just one thing different. His breath don't smell like liquor, but he's drunk all right, and I've seen plenty of 'em back in Tennessee but I never thought the day'd come when I'd have to come and tell you or anybody else that Jim Robert's drinkin'."

The preacher was aghast, incredulous, and said so.

"Jim Robert can't be drinkin'. He's my right hand man in the church. Together we've prayed mightily over the evils of rum. He's no drinkin' sinner."

"Then, preacher," said Ella Mae, "You be at our house this evenin' about five forty-five when Jim Robert gets home and you can see for yourself. Jim Robert says that he ain't had a drink in his life, but the way he has trouble keepin' on the sidewalk even, you jus' know that somebody's givin' him liquor on the way home."

The preacher was at Jim Robert's house before five forty-five, sitting out on the front porch. Jim Robert came staggering up, displaying all of those characteristics of the mildly inebriated that lead women to cross over to the other side of the path and grandmothers to call playing children from off the sidewalk. Jim Robert, a little unoriented but unlike the shamefaced, common drunk, joyfully came up to the preacher, slapped him a little too hard on the back, made a few remarks that were not quite reverential.

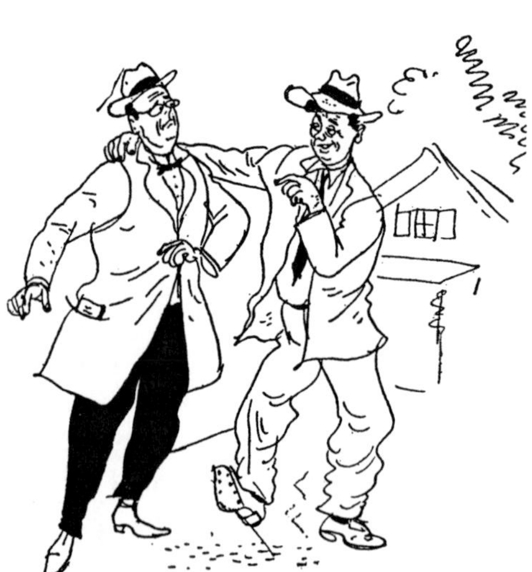

To himself the preacher was saying, "This is bad. This will have to be investigated. We shall probably have to turn Brother Stevens out of the church."

The preacher stayed for supper but there was possibility that tears were mixed with dishwater. Ella Mae's supper was not quite up to perfection, and no wonder. Jim Robert had taken to drinking. Even the preacher knew it. A little after supper Jim Robert "sobered up." There was no berating, no adroit questioning, just a lot of stunned uncertainty. The preacher went home.

In the same block of the city in which the preacher lived, also lived the physician of the plant where Jim Robert worked. The doctor was not of the preacher's flock but they were friendly. The next day the troubled minister of the gospel went in the evening to the home of that person, who, in the lingo of many shops, is called "The Castor Oil Artist." The preacher poured out his apprehensions.

"Doctor, one of my church members works at your plant. He is a valuable church member, as undoubtedly he is a valuable worker. For a long while he has been the very emblem of sobriety. He's loathed liquor and has preached against it. Now it seems that through some queer turn of affairs he's becomin' a drunkard. His wife is frightened because every afternoon when he returns from work he's offensively intoxicated. Only last evening I saw him in that pitiful state. Could you, Doctor, confidentially of course, look around a bit at the plant and give me the benefit of what you learn. Maybe he's drinkin' on the job. On a time basis he gets home just at the hour he always has, and he doesn't get out of the shop any earlier. He doesn't have time to do any drinkin' unless he drinks out of a bottle on the way home. It's all very distressin', doctor. Will you help us?"

The doctor promised. "Come back here tomorrow night at eight o'clock," he said. "I will have all day tomorrow to make inquiries."

The preacher and the doctor met the next night as arranged. The doctor was not hilarious, but he acted as though he thought the preacher ought to be hilarious. The preacher should have been, because the great burden had shifted from the preacher's shoulder to the doctor's.

Here is what the doctor said. "Your man Stevens had not been drinking liquor. You can get that off your mind. You can get it off his wife's mind. At least, there is no sign of his drinking liquor, but he has been drunk all right, drunk over and over. He has been drunk every night for weeks. I've slipped up on my job, not you. Here's how it happens.

"Stevens is a metal degreaser. He works on a 'tri' degreaser. Degreasing is not done in liquid trichlorethylene but only in its vapors. Unless the machine is working perfectly, some vapors get out and 'tri' vapors have a very queer effect. Almost like alcohol, this pleasant industrial chemical breathed in by any worker leads to a state of exotic euphoria, to hilarity, to a staggering gait, to a twisted tongue. More than that, just like alcohol, some workers get addicted to these 'tri jags.' Slowly, and without awareness, workers take on a love for the exhilaration that 'tri' brings. They become 'tri' happy. Funny stuff, this 'tri.'

"Today, thanks to you, sir, we found a small leak in Stevens' degreasing machine. How long he has been breathing 'tri' God only knows. Just enough of those vapors to make him 'high' by the end of the work day. No wonder his wife thought he was drunk. No wonder you thought he was drunk. He was drunk, but not with liquor. Today we plugged up that leak, and nobody will be able to get these cheap 'jags' any more. Real drinks cost money, but maybe you wouldn't know about that, preacher."

Jim Robert was not "turned out" of church. In fact, there are now plans to make him a deacon. If you have no place for your worship, we commend to you that church to which Jim Robert and Ella Mae are ardently devoted, but don't be suspicious of Jim Robert. He was never drunk in his life—on liquor.

Chapter 42

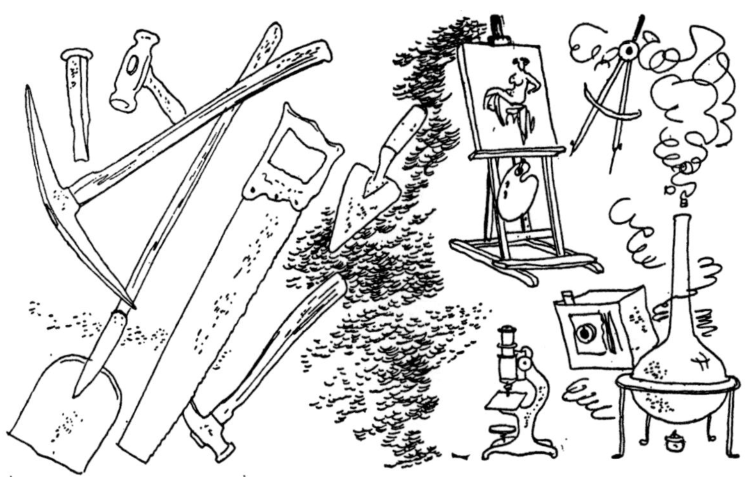

The Preferred Professions

ALREADY I am committed to inability to separate professions from other occupations. At all times the nod will be made to the portrait painter, but he is the archetype for the photographer. In turn, the photographer is the archetype for the blueprint maker. Let's not again go all through that maze. By any grouping of workers there are small numbers representing the higher callings in life. They have their plagues too. Banish the idea that the diseases of work are limited to those whose implements are the pick and shovel, the hammer and chisel, the brush and trowel, the caliper and tachometer.

The most variedly exposed man of all professions is the chemist — working with his creations of undisclosed toxicity, the deviser of many substances that later prove to be the newer hazards, working not with one or two materials at a time, but, instead, possibly a hundred. All of the dangers from chemicals shared by industry are recapitulated, at least in miniature, in the laboratory of the chemist.

This is no new concept. Chaucer in one of his tales causes the alchemist to describe his sorry plight after his chemical efforts to find the Philosopher's Stone. He says:

> "Al that I hadde, I have y-lost thereby;
> And god wot, so hath many mo than I.
> Ther I was wont to be right fresh and gay
> Of clothing and of other good array,
> Now may I were an hose upon myn heed;
> And wher my colour was bothe fresh and reed,
> Now is it wan and of a leden hewe;
> Who-so it useth, sore shal he rewe.
> And of my swink yet blered is myn ye."

Every other chemist may make his own contributions descriptive of his own woes.

Assuming that medicine, despite court decisions, may be a profession, its devotees may suffer any of a multitude of professional afflictions. Only one may be mentioned.

Among roentgenologists, or, if you prefer, radiologists, sterility is common. Cast about you and count the number of children of your friends among the roentgenologists. If they be fairly old, if they have long been in the specialty of roentgenology, if they were roentgenologists during that period of their life when the begetting of children is usual, the greater number will prove by your count to be childless. As I write, I count on my fingers twelve x-ray workers, all of whom are without sons or daughters. The property of the x-ray is to destroy both in men and women those cells necessary in the reproduction of life. Protection may be afforded—yes. In recent years, protection has been so improved that sterility is not the rule. Nearly every normal man and woman crave children of their own bodies. In the case of this one class of physicians, this craving may be unsatisfied because of one of the doctor's occupational ills.

Over and over, I, as an industrial hygienist, have acquired in mild fashion the very diseases that I have been investigating. The day's work may have called for a study of a brass foundry, only to be followed by a night of brass founder's chills. Testing for carbon tetrachloride, this chemical has laid me low, thus furnishing better proof to me than any instrument that dangerous quantities prevailed. Studying arc welding, short wave ultra-violet light has produced half-blindness, ruining any opportunity for full work during the next two or three days. Without my goodwill and without any desire, there have been times nearly every month when I suffered from a different occupational disease. If these experiences have served any good purpose, it has been to make me more sympathetic with those workers day by day exposed to injurious substances.

Close by the physician stands the nurse. Any communicable disease which she may acquire in her work becomes an occupational disease. If you acquire scarlet fever from some unknown exposure, into no ranks of an occupational disease does your case fall; let the nurse who ministers to you acquire your scarlet fever, then this becomes an occupational affair for her.

By this time possibly you are trying to bring forth the school teacher as an exception — then I thwart you by painting your school teacher standing before the blackboard, eraser in one hand, orange colored chalk in the other. For years, but not necessarily at this time, orange, yellow, lemon and divers other colored crayons have depended upon lead chromates for their pigments. It is not recorded that any lead poisoning cases have arisen from this source, but here is the theoretical exposure that, on occasion, might be consummated in clinical lead poisoning in a teacher.

When I was a medical student and in the dissecting room, a popular and able instructor resigned. Some of us planned a petition, urging him to remain, at least throughout our period of anatomical training. Selfishness made us unconcerned about oncoming groups of students. The professor in charge heard of our plan and admonished.

"It will do no good to send in a petition. This man is necessarily leaving. He has become sensitized to the chemicals used in the treatment of cadavers. Any contact with a body in the dissecting room is followed by violent skin inflammation — you must have seen his bandaged arms. For his own good, he must go."

Go into the photographer's dark room. On his shelves you will find such chemicals as these — pyrogallic acid, metol, hydroquinone, sodium sulfide, diamidophenol (amidol), rodinal, gold chloride, citric acid, bromide compounds, bichromates, hydroxides, mineral acids, silver compounds, picric acid, alcohols, acetates, mercury, salts, formaldehyde, cyanogen compounds, benzol, anilin compounds, etc. All of them and more are enemies of the photographer's skin. Some are well known as common causes of dermatitis.

In all of life, the engineer is ubiquitous. One of him may be found directing explosive firing in a mine, another supervising the manufacture of chemicals, a third drawing plans for a new skyscraper, a fourth scheming for safer traffic. In industry, wherever occupational disease exposures prevail, one or more engineers are likely to be included in those exposed. Let one engineer tell his own medical history, much as he told it to me.

"I'm one of the engineers building the hydro-electric dam down on the Setan River. I am sick, Doctor, and my wife and children are sick. We're all pretty badly shaken. It must be something communicable. I got it first, and then quickly one child after another, and then my wife. We have frightful headaches, just as though something was on the inside of our heads boring out. At times I have been willing to dash my head against a stone wall, be-

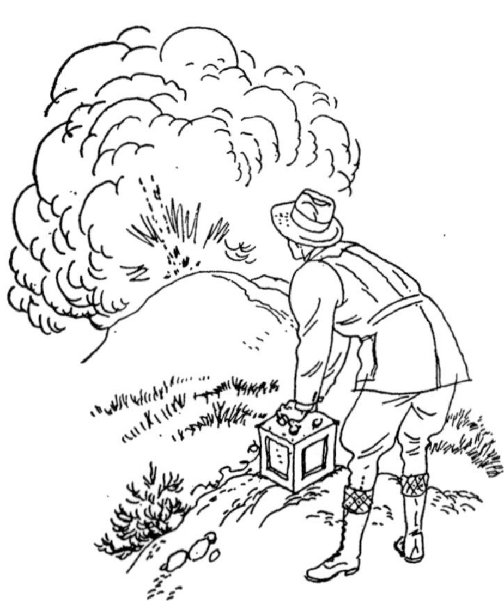

lieving that there would be less pain from the outside than came from the inside. This has been pretty hard on the children. At the same time, our hearts beat very fast. I am not a doctor, but I can count pulse, and our heartbeats are so fast at times that I can't count them. They must run at times 140 or 150. I took our temperatures with the thermometer, but everyone of us was perfectly normal. What is this all about? I think maybe we all have meningitis or infantile paralysis."

Since other members of the household were involved, for the moment I was off guard and did not expect an occupational disease, but as part of the routine questions I inquired,

"What is your particular work at the dam?"

Back came the illuminating reply, "I'm the firing boss. I supervise all of the drilling for explosion shots; I'm in charge of the dynamite dump, I supervise the loading of all firing holes and the placing of fuse wires."

Then came my inquiry, "Have you been at this work long?"

"No," the engineer replied, "only for a few months. The old boss retired just before this new contract started. I had been in the cost estimating department for years and was in line for a promotion. This new job is a real advance for me."

By this time I believed I knew the answer, but it would have been foolish to have jumped to a conclusion. There were many more questions, examinations, visits with the engineer's wife and children. Then came the diagnosis.

"You have a 'dynamite head.' Your headaches come from the explosives at your work. Every explosive worker is apt to have this experience. You are fairly new, not yet enough experienced."

The incredulous engineer said, "That's foolish, Doctor, my wife and children aren't engineers. They don't come around the dam more than once a month."

"No, it isn't foolish. On your clothing you carry enough powder dust to your home two or three times a week to bowl them over with the same disease. With you it is a disease of the trade. For them that is not so — it is just a disease that father brings home."

"Maybe you're right, Doctor, but what can we do about it?"

"Well, sir, there is a strange thing about dynamite. When it is around you all the time, you don't have the disease. Seemingly, intermittent exposure is necessary. I'm telling you what to do. Slip two or three grains of powder under your hat-band and forget about them. Take a few more grains and safely hide them about the house. The chances are there won't be any more headaches."

And so it all worked out, but several days later back came the engineer. "Doctor, my family and I are all right now. We're cured, but everybody that calls on us at my house gets a hell of a headache. What are we going to do about that?"

And now I was at the end of my row.

"Possibly," I proposed, "you ought to go back to being the cost accountant engineer."

That stung just a little. He went away sorrowfully.

One by one, most of the remaining professions might be associated with some opportunity for health impairment. Only a few groups escape, such as the jurists, the lawyers, the bankers, and the office executives.

Then, over and above the professions there may be a group of people who are the drones, the idlers, the clippers of coupons, the livers on inheritances — they have no profession. But let it be remembered that having no occupation is the worst of all occupational diseases.

Chapter 43

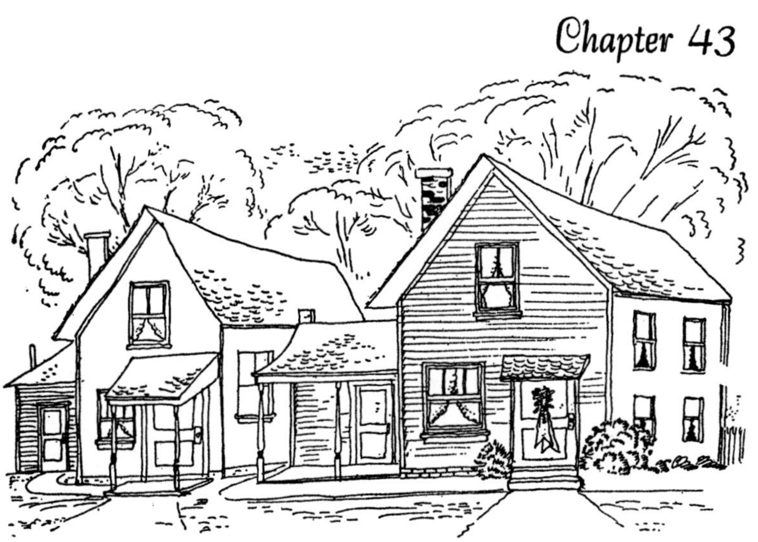

Chrysanthemums' Fingerprints

A BABY died next door — died from pneumonia — from broncho-pneumonia. "Next door" in this instance means next door to another city residence where a needy family during the life-burning years of the depression scorned "relief" and eked out a precarious economic security through a petty business carried out in the basement, in the dining room, and garage. That family made insect powder.

"Bad blood" long had marked the relations of the two families — even before the baby was born. The baby's family, a little more prosperous than the insecticide family, felt that the whole neighborhood was being blighted when one household was turned into a factory.

After the funeral, the irate father instituted what was probably an "abatement of nuisance suit," claiming that some poison from the insect powder had killed the baby. The judge made a commendable temporary ruling. This called upon the city department of health to investigate the matter. If any proof might be furnished that any appreciable quantity of the insect powder in fact reached the next door home, an order of abatement would be issued; otherwise not.

I was called upon to make this investigation functioning as I was, as the head of one public health department, but particularly was I chosen because many years earlier I was the discoverer, or more rightly, the rediscoverer of this particular insecticide as a marked skin irritant.

At the home of the offending family, I was admitted by a frightened, discouraged old lady, who was utterly amazed that anybody might believe her insecticides could harm anyone, even a baby, in another house eighteen feet away. She was particularly grieved that the complaints against her had been given wide newspaper publicity. She sobbed, "The whole city is down on me."

She was the widow of the man who had started this home business years before. At his death, she had assumed responsibility along with a son and daughter. The two children peddled the insecticide while the widow, staying at home, filled packages, sealed openings, stuck on labels and posted the little ledger showing the losses or occasional profits. Her story was a simple one:

"We only make one insect powder. It is the same kind that hundreds of other people make and sell over the country. It is pyrethrum insect powder. Pyrethrum, you know, is just ground-up chrysanthemum buds. My husband before me did just as we do now. We buy the chrysanthemum buds already ground up in fifty pound cans. All we do is to mix about half with some other powder like wood meal. The pyrethrum by itself would be too strong. We don't have any machinery to stir up dust and there is never more than three or four of us working here in the house and then only once in a while when we are mixing and when we get a lot of orders. I don't see how anybody could blame us. All that we're trying to do is to make a living. None of my folks want to go on relief. We feel that the only difference between going to the poorhouse and going on relief is that when you go on relief you just bring the poorhouse to your house. Do you think that we are mean and wicked and baby-killing folks, Doctor?"

"No, Mrs. Simpson. I can't imagine you ever having done a vicious thing in your whole life. It is rather heartening to see anybody at your age willing to work so hard to make your own way in the world, but we must be sure that you are not harming any of the neighbors. The Board of Health has ample authority to demand the abatement of any nuisance. There is no sure way in the world of proving that the dead baby was injured by dusts from your pyrethrum, but if we should find any pyrethrum in the baby's house, you may be called on to give up this work in a residential district."

You wouldn't expect chrysanthemums to be the ready cause of a disease — not those lovely chrysanthemums that make a football crowd look like a Paisley shawl. Truly those varieties of chrysanthemums are innocuous, but other types seemingly have a grudge against mankind.

In 1921, I stumbled upon pyrethrum dermatitis. That year, one of the opportunities given me by industry for scientific investigation was concerned with a plant that scarcely may be associated with any well identified industry. The organization bottled castor oil, flavoring extracts and catsup, made peanut butter, patent medicine and insecticides, and ground mustard. Self-styled, this plant was labeled "Manufacturing Chemists."

One product was an insecticide in powder form, packaged in small tricornate cardboard bellows. Blown about the habitat of insects, the powder was undeniably efficacious. It was prepared in a small section of the factory, a department employing some eighty-odd workers. During the summer months many of these men and women developed a disturbing skin disease in the elbow folds, at the shoe tops, around the neck, or on the upper eyelids. The work operation was a dusty one, and it seemed obvious that dust settling on these parts and leached out by perspiration was causing the trouble. We who were conducting the investigation reached this conclusion immediately, but the management scoffed emphatically.

"All we're doing is grinding up chrysanthemum buds," they pointed out. "You can't expect an ordinary garden flower to be the cause of all this trouble."

The expectation was not merely sustained, but supported.

Through many decades, much of the romance of Dalmatia has been linked with its broad fields of Dalmatian daisies. For years, the buds of this variety of chrysanthemum have constituted an outstanding portion of the province's industry. Prose and poetry have portrayed the beauty of this flower, but not divulged is the secret that, hidden within its petals, is a potent irritant. Although Dalmatia gave name to "Dalmatian Insect Powder," the world's commercial supplies are in part obtained from Persia, the Caucasus, Montenegro, and Japan. California, likewise, has been found to have a climate favorable to the luxurious growth of the plant, and is a notable commercial source.

Lest the uninitiated form the opinion that this material represents only a chemical curiosity, let it be recorded that in so remote a year as 1917, one million five hundred and four thousand pounds were imported into the United States in bales, most likely to have been labeled "Buhach," since this is its favorite name in many portions of the globe.

Wavering just a little, the management called in its own plant engineer to make installations eliminating some of the dustiness of the operation. Promptly he acquired the disease, which rather crystallized our own belief as to the cause. Unconvinced, a junior member of the management entered the department to give a demonstration of the complete innocuousness of the company's product. He amply coated himself with fine pyrethrum, and promptly developed the worst dermatitis of all. The already afflicted workers concealed their sadistic delight in this instance only a little less than a flock of floating barrage balloons.

This painful approach to conviction proved distressing. Such a state of sensitivity was created in the young official that he confided years later, "All I had to do after that was merely walk into the department, touching nothing, then get my hat and start for the hospital. Time after time every inch of my skin was involved, so that I peeled off even the skin of my palms."

When publication was made concerning the investigation, it was

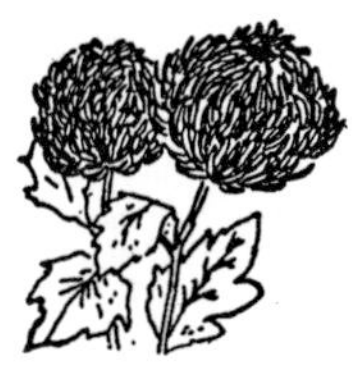

hailed as disclosing a new disease. Fortunately my name was not associated with it, that fashion having long since been discarded. Indeed, just the opposite happened: for years thereafter, within that small group of the brotherhood given to the use of first names, I was dubbed "Pyrethrum McCord." My name was not attached to the disease, but the disease name was attached to mine.

Leaping over nearly two decades from 1921 back to Mrs. Simpson's house I found that much dust settled about on shelves, ledges, furniture and window sills. Obviously, this partly was vegetable dust, but I was hard put to devise any test that might prove beyond peradventure that any of this same dust reached the neighboring house. I conceived the plan of collecting all possible dust from the neighboring house, extracting this and attempting to isolate pyrethrotoxic acid, one of the active constituents of pyrethrum, but the chemists shook their heads horizontally. Then the obvious plan came to mind. Chrysanthemum flowers undoubtedly have pollen granules. These would be as characteristic as fingerprints. I would seek out the particular pollen type of pyrethrum, would look for the granules in the two houses. If found in Mrs. Simpson's house, and not found in the neighbor's, the old lady would be in the clear. If found in abundance in both houses, she faced an end to her business. Pollen granules were destined to settle this neighborhood row.

Under the microscope, to my discomfiture, were dozens of kinds of pollen granules. I recognized a few of our old friends, such as ragweed, but I had no microscopic acquaintance with pyrethrum. One particular variety was overwhelmingly numerous. I guessed these would be pyrethrum, but, in science, guessing is taboo. It was necessary to establish the identity of pyrethrum's specific granules. I went to the botanists. They seemed to be on speaking terms with every pollen imaginable, save pyrethrum. One by one they eased out of range. Then I went to the library. After examining more than a score of books, I found it — a perfect picture of pyrethrum's pollen — enlarged many times. The granule was the one that dominated my own microscopic fields. Now I was ready to make the crucial test.

Back at the neighbor's house, with squirrel-hair brushes, which the public for some unknown reason calls camel-hair brushes, I made little piles of dusts from the nursery, from the floor crevices, from the mantlepiece, from the window casings.

By this time I hoped that I would find no pyrethrum. Personally, I was on Mrs. Simpson's side, but scientifically I was non-partisan.

Under the microscope, there they were, numbers of them, unmistakable, unhidable proof that Mrs. Simpson's pyrethrum had been blown next door.

At the offices of the Board of Health first I made my report orally and later in writing. The Commissioner shook his head and said, "Looks like we'll have an abatement order."

"Commissioner," I said, "Don't do anything for a couple of days. Maybe I can handle this without legal action."

Seated with Mrs. Simpson in her dusty dining room, made over into her workroom, I held back all accounts that possibly after all she might have contributed to the infant's death.

Instead I said, "Mrs. Simpson, you're pretty much cooped up here in the city. At least one neighbor has complained about you, and some of the others are getting suspicious. How much better off you'd be carrying on your little business out in the country. You could do the work there just as well or even better, and there'll be no neighbors to point fingers of accusation in your direction. I know just the place, thirty-eight acres, plenty of room for everything. How would you like to move?"

Mrs. Simpson did move, taking her cans of pyrethrum with her. The business goes on. If you are ever in need of pyrethrum insect powder, I would like to recommend Mrs. Simpson's particular brand. It contains at least some pyrethrum, for I have identified it by its peculiar pollen granules.

Chapter 44

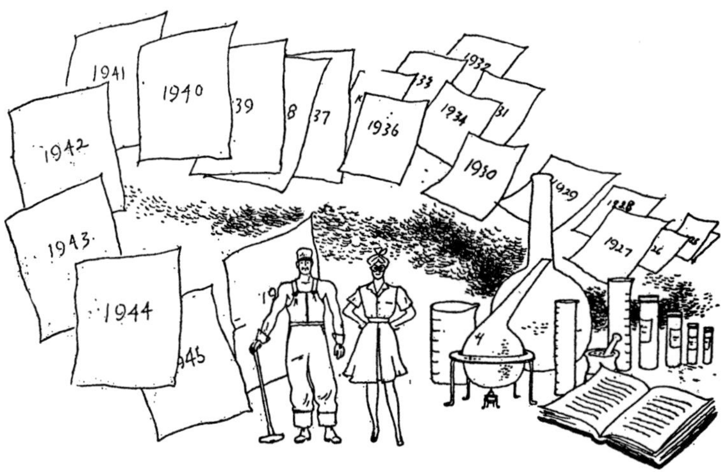

This Amazing Present

With shameless disregard for the niceties of chronology, I have darted back and forth through twenty-five years of industrial hygiene. With equal disregard for special orientation, unmapped leaps have been made from Canada to Panama without checking off the mile posts. Only disservice to the reader could have issued from a stodgy diary that noted among a thousand entries that in June, 1924, I was puttering in a white lead factory in Ohio; that in August, 1933, my days and some nights were spent in a sand mine in Missouri; that December of 1942 found me in Michigan, participating in the building of military tanks for the crushing of the affronting wicked.

Even more unexciting might have been any bracketing that nicely assorted me into the laboratory technician, the research investigator, the university professor, the writer of all too many technical brochures, the occupant of the witness chair, and the consultant. With unhidden selfish concern, I am mindful that, for decades yet uncalendered, I may have to live with this book. You are not so committed.

In lieu of the orderly and the documentary, I have sought to beguile you into a tour of the booths of a personal industrial hygienic state fair. As a substitute for the biggest potatoes, the smallest dust particles have been placed on exhibition; prize winning pumpkin pies and jellies have given way to irritant greases and oils; blue ribbon stock have yielded their stalls to blue ribbon men and women workers, who without the workings of industrial hygiene might not now be in the lands of the living.

But no figurative display of these formative years captivates like the dazzling present.

Now the pioneer days of industrial hygiene are over. Now industrial hygiene is a part of public health, politics, labor union contracts, trade association agenda, insurance company enterprises and the trading stock of legislators — as much a part of some plant management as cost accounting or salvage.

The little handful of five or six physicians of 1919 and an equal number of engineers who called themselves industrial hygienists were indeed not the founders or creators of industrial hygiene. At most, we were the human repository of the hereditary genes passed on by Ramazzini.

Attesting the fecundity of this little group sprawled over the nation is the fact that twenty-five years later, by 1944, industrial hygienists were so numerous that a national body had been brought into being, with officers, directors, by-laws, blocs and controversies. Federal and state departments now squabble among themselves as to which shall have the honor and glory, but particularly the appropriations, for safeguarding the workers' health. Insurance companies, with the "safety first" movement as a lucrative precedent for cutting down claims, have taken to industrial hygiene as similarly promising. A few political campaigns have been waged on promises of more and better occupational disease legislation. Some labor unions have made the discovery that an effective appeal to be made to membership is the assurance of work places free from direful exposures. High school boys contemplate industrial hygiene as a possible career, along with such other choices as electrical engineering, law, teaching or football coaching. In brief, the protection of the health of the worker has been integrated into American life. Shades of that cold morning traveling on an open handcar to our first job!

If any member of our little band possessed any awareness that later on he would be earmarked as a maker of industrial hygiene history, no sign of this raised its head. Nor have we been. Occasionally, though, maybe we did get a look over the hill to this present time when industrial hygiene is taken for granted.

Struggling through scrawny years seeking understanding, we may have had our own subconscious Cinderella complex that in some future day borne on our own shoulders, industrial hygiene would be delivered to a needy and appreciative world in a golden panoply. Whatever happened, we were not the accoucheurs. The real forces that created industrial hygiene's present heyday largely were accidental.

The depression years beginning in 1929 brought to light hundreds of workmen, with or without impaired health from work, who were entirely willing to sue employers on the flimsiest of pretexts. Frightened industry, long little concerned in occupational diseases and industrial hygiene, began a loud clamor for protection, for legislation for the safeguarding of its plants. Touched in the pocketbook, industrial management became the great sponsor for industrial hygiene. A suing workman in the absence of any occupational disease legislation might demand fifty thousand dollars damages and by a jury might be awarded fifteen, twenty-five or thirty thousand dollars — seldom the full amount, but under the orderly processes of state-supervised occupational disease compensation, awards even for deaths seldom would exceed six thousand dollars. Hence the speedy metamorphosis of many manufacturers into pleaders for legislative protection.

Harking to the demands of industrialists, chorused by labor organizations with a slightly different lay, there came an outpouring of Federal moneys for the protection of the health of the workers. Most states have set up Bureaus of Industrial Hygiene or Occupational Disease Prevention. An array of chemists, engineers, physicians, public health workers, almost overnight emerged as industrial hygienists. The protection of the worker was discovered to be a public function, and well may it be so regarded.

The high status of industrial hygiene as it is today has resulted more from the dramatic appeal of a few startling happenings in industry than all of the combined efforts of that small number of us who anointed ourselves with some feeling of developmental proprietorship. When a few cases of disastrous radium poisoning occurred on the Atlantic seaboard a few years ago, industrial hygiene then and there was groomed for a stellar role. When the catastrophe of Gauley Bridge became known to the public in its full tragedy, industrial hygiene, already knighted, approached deification. Such spectacular occupational disease outbreaks were industrial hygiene's springboards.

Then came war, and the field of the cloth of gold for the conservation of the worker's health. Whatever handicaps may have been thrown around an orderly development of the protection of this country's workers, all were swept aside by the feverish programs of national preservation. On all sides, were heard endless variations of the statement that industrial production is the heart of warfare and worker protection is the heart of production. The health of workers assumed new values. No longer was emphasis limited to the avoidance of suffering, the curtailment of the work span of the tradesman as an individual or the elimination of unnecessary compensation and medical bills. The individual worker took on national importance — the wheels of his machine must continually turn, not for his wage or the profit of his employer, but that the nation might survive.

"Not just once does the ox need his tail to brush away the flies," runs an old Creole proverb. Not just once does the nation need a worker to assemble a machine gun, to build a rifle, to construct an ambulance, to shape a soldier's cot, to weave a blanket. Tomorrow and next day his trained hands even more may be required. Industrial hygiene is in full flower.

Come war, come peace — new machines, chemicals, processes and products continually will attend industry. New and direful dangers will replace old ones. Cunning means have been found to circumvent or banish the evil qualities of unwanted work conditions in the past. Even more acceptable devices and procedures will be created to meet the requirements of coming years. Better skilled and abler men will rise up to meet these newer threats to the worker's health and to keep in force and improve upon those measures now applied. Industrial hygiene will move toward exactness as a science.

New groups of industrial workers will apply for employment in factories, mills, mines, and shops. Always manpower will be needed. In a coming day they will be even more adequately safeguarded, until in time no work will be associated with any prospective, unwanted toll of the worker's well-being.

This has been the hope and the plan from the beginning.

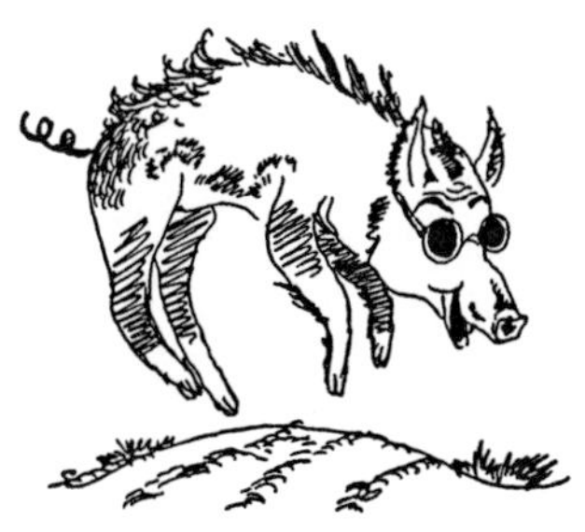

LaVergne, TN USA
11 April 2011
223723LV00004B/9/A

9 781930 665200